J. K. Ransley · J. K. Donnelly · N. W. Read (Eds.)
Food and Nutritional Supplements

Springer
Berlin
Heidelberg
New York
Barcelona
Hong Kong
London
Milan
Paris
Singapore
Tokyo

J. K. Ransley · J. K. Donnelly · N. W. Read (Eds.)

Food and Nutritional Supplements

Their Role in Health and Disease

With 13 Figures and 24 Tables

Springer

Joan K. Ransley and Dr. Judith K. Donnelly
Public Health Nutrition Unit
Trinity and All Saints
College of the University of Leeds
Leeds LS18 5HD, UK

Professor Nicholas W. Read
The Centre for Integrated Medicine
Institute for General Practice and Primary Care
University of Sheffield
Northern General Hospital
Sheffield S5 7AU, UK

ISBN 3-540-41737-0 Springer-Verlag Berlin Heidelberg New York

Library of Congress Cataloging-in-Publication Data

Food and nutritional supplements : their role in health and disease / J. Ransley,
J. Donnelly, N. Read (eds.)
p. cm.
Includes bibliographical references and index.
ISBN 3540417370 (alk. paper)
1. Dietary supplements. 2. Nutrition. I. Ransley, J. (Joan), 1955- II. Donnelly, J. (Judith),
1958- III. Read, N.W.

RM258.5 .F66 2001
613.2--dc21

Springer-Verlag Berlin Heidelberg New York
a member of BertelsmannSpringer Science+Business Media GmbH

http://www.springer.de

Printed in Germany

The figure for the coverdesign was originally produced by Osiris, Leeds, UK.

Typesetting: Fotosatz-Service Köhler GmbH, Würzburg
Coverdesign: design & production, Heidelberg

Printed on acid-free paper SPIN: 10761404 52/3020mh – 5 4 3 2 1 0

Preface

What This Book is About

It is estimated that 40% of people in the UK take nutritional supplements. This statistic has risen dramatically in recent years and is predicted to increase further over the next five years. Across the whole of Western Europe the market for these products is also growing. Consumers have been encouraged to take more responsibility for their own health and this has resulted in the use in self medication facilated by changes in the regulations controlling the sale and distribution of medicines. The purpose of this book is to examine the phenomenon of self-medication with nutritional supplements from both a biological and a psychological perspective. The book begins by discussing the range of supplements and their markets. There is also a consideration of why health professionals need to know about the efficacy or otherwise of food and nutritional supplements, and how the need for particular nutrients varies throughout the life span. Chapters on vitamin B_6, folic acid, phyto-oestrogens and pre- and probiotics examine the scientific basis for supplementation and evidence for efficacy in health and disease states. The topics were selected to illustrate controversial issues surrounding diet and the use of supplementation in health and disease. Effective healing and prevention of ill health does not only depend on the biological action of a product but on how much faith the consumer invests. This book also examines how confidence in a particular supplement can regulate the psychobiological mechanisms responsible for maintaining healthy responses to life situations and discusses the moral dilemma posed by selling psychological regulators in the guise of biologically active substances. This book will be of particular interest to pharmacists, dietitians, nutritionists, nurses, psychologists and workers in the food and drug industries and anybody who is concerned about food and health.

Introduction

As nutritionists we embrace the idea that to eat well is to live well. Eating well is a good starting point for a life that is not only physically healthy but also socially and psychologically balanced. From this perspective the ever increasing consumption of food and nutritional supplements over the last decade is an alarming phenomenon that tells us how insecure people feel about their health and well being. Pharmacies, drug stores, health food shops and supermarkets all stock a vast array of preparations which include vitamins, minerals, oils derived from flowers and fish, tonics and herbal products. These preparations are also readily available by mail order and purchase over the Internet.

Why is it that so many people feel the need to take these products? What guidance are they given about taking them? Are they safe? Do they make any measurable difference to how people feel? Are they effective in preventing serious disease? Is there really a good case for taking supplements or will a healthy diet provide all that is required to optimise health and prevent disease?

Most people obtain information about nutritional supplements from articles in popular magazines and newspapers but it is health professionals such as family doctors, practice nurses and pharmacists who field their more searching questions on the efficacy and safety of these preparations in the prevention and treatment of disease. Family doctors, nurses and pharmacists are all well qualified health professionals but they are hard pressed to keep abreast of the new research on the complex role nutrients play in the aetiology, prevention and treatment of human disease. Pharmacists are in a particularly important position in this regard since, like the apothecaries of old, they have a dual role in giving advice to patients and selling food and nutritional supplements. Pharmacies remain the most popular retail outlet from which supplements are sold. Market research has shown time and time again that it is the presence of a pharmacist that gives added value to pharmaceutical products and encourages the consumer to trust and buy the products on the shelves of the pharmacy. Family doctors also need to have an informed dialogue with their patients, many of whom possess firm convictions about taking supplements for specific conditions such as rheumatoid arthritis, premenstrual tension or for nebulous, less well defined states such as feeling tired and run down.

As the popularity of these products is rising exponentially and conflicting reports on their use continue to hit the headlines, all health professionals are called upon increasingly to provide a well balanced opinion on their efficacy and safety. Health professionals need to be as well informed as they can on such matters. This is the reason for writing this book. The experts who have contributed chapters are actively engaged in research into the science underpinning the complex role nutrients have in the human body and each chapter addresses a key theme of relevance to evaluating the role food and nutritional supplements play in human health.

The book is organised into three main sections. The first section sets the scene and outlines the phenomenal growth in the market for food and nutritional supplements over recent years. It also explains why the body's need for nutrients varies over the lifecycle and during the course of an illness or during trauma. A chapter argues the case for extending the knowledge base of health professionals in the field of nutrition. Another chapter explains why patients may feel the need to self medicate with supplements which may have little biological effect but fulfil a patients need to believe in a substance which can relieve their suffering. In short, this chapter examines the role of good and nutritional supplements as placebos. The second part of the book examines the science behind the role key nutrients and components in food can play in the aetiology, prevention and treatment of disease. Vitamin B_6, folic acid, antioxidants, phytoestrogens, pre and probiotics are all considered in detail here. The final section, evaluates by way of example, two common disease states for which nutrients and components in food can play a role in prevention and treatment- these are, coronary heart disease and rheumatoid arthritis. These two conditions lie high on the agenda of patient worries and concerns about their health.

Each of the contributors has provided a comprehensive yet concise coverage of the latest developments in our understanding of aspects of nutrition in relation to food and nutritional supplements. We have aimed to give the reader insights into the phenomenon of self medication with dietary supplements and why consumers are willing to invest so much time, money and belief in the efficacy of this over the counter healthcare sector. We hope this book will provide facts and remove some of the mystique about supplements and provide the reader with an informed view from which to base judgements when making decisions about healthy eating and the use of dietary supplements.

August 2000 *Joan K. Ransley, Judith K. Donnelly, Nicholas W. Read*

Acknowledgements

We would like to thank our colleagues in the nutrition world for both contributing to the chapters in this book and for helping us to make such a success of the conference *Nutrition for Pharmacists* held in 1999 at Trinity and All Saints College, Leeds. We would also like to thank Springer-Verlag for their enthusiasm in encouraging us to produce this book as a result of the conference. In particular we would like to thank Mathew Joynson for undertaking the original research in preparation for the conference, Sonja Pos and Sylvia Simpson for their help in preparing this book.

Announcement

It is with deep regret that we record the death of one of our authors, Professor Anthony Diplock earlier this year. His chapter ***Antioxidants, nutrition and health*** *is* a fitting memorial to his ground breaking work on free radicals and the role of antioxidants in health.

Contents

1 The Rise and Rise of Food and Nutritional Supplements – an Overview of the Market
Joan K. Ransley . . . 1

1.1 Introduction . . . 1

1.2 The Products . . . 1

1.3 What are People Taking? . . . 2
1.3.1 Cod Liver Oil . . . 2
1.3.2 Multivitamins . . . 3
1.3.3 Single Vitamins . . . 3
1.3.4 Evening Primrose Oil . . . 3
1.3.5 Minerals . . . 4
1.3.6 Garlic Products . . . 4
1.3.7 Functional Foods . . . 4

1.4 Growth Across Western Europe . . . 5

1.5 Who Manufactures Vitamin, Mineral and Dietary Supplements? 6

1.6 Retail Distribution of Vitamins, Minerals and Dietary Supplements . . . 6

1.7 What is Driving the Growth in this Market? . . . 7
1.7.1 Age and Lifestyle Trends Spin the Market . . . 8
1.7.2 The Trend Towards Self-Medication . . . 9
1.7.2.1 Concerns About Illness Drive Demand . . . 9
1.7.2.2 Changes in the Pharmacy . . . 10
1.7.2.3 Changes in Primary Health Care . . . 10

1.8 Do Supplement Users Need to Take Supplements? . . . 11

1.9 Regulating the Market . . . 12

1.10 The Future for Vitamins, Minerals and Dietary Supplements . . . 14

1.11 Conclusion . . . 15

1.12 References . . . 15

2 **Why do Health Professionals Need to Know More About Nutrition?**
Matthew E. Joynson . . . 17

2.1 Introduction . . . 17
2.1.1 The Implication of Diet in Disease . . . 17

2.2 Our Hunger for Knowledge . . . 18

2.3 Health Professionals: the Authorative Source of Nutrition Information? . . . 19

2.4 Nutrition: the Orphan Discipline . . . 21

2.5 What are the Obstacles to Giving Nutrition Advice? . . . 22

2.6 The Updated Role of Health Professionals: a New Approach . . . 23
2.6.1 Tailored Dietary Advice . . . 23
2.6.2 Different People, Different Dietary Needs . . . 24
2.6.3 Drug-Nutrient Interactions . . . 25
2.6.4 The Impact of Diet in Health Economics . . . 25

2.7 Conclusion . . . 26

2.8 References . . . 27

3 **Nutrient Requirements in Health and Disease**
Judith K. Donnelly . . . 29

3.1 Introduction . . . 29

3.2 What Nutrients are Needed, and How Much? . . . 29

3.3 Dietary Reference Values . . . 30

3.4 Meeting the Targets . . . 30

3.5 Pregnancy and Lactation – Life-Long Health Implications of Nutrition . . . 32

3.6 The Weaning Process . . . 35

3.7 Childhood . . . 36

3.8 Younger Schoolchildren . . . 38

3.9 Adolescence . . . 38

3.10 Adulthood . . . 39

3.11 Older Years . . . 40

3.12 Conclusion . . . 42

3.13 References . . . 43

4 **Placebo and Panacea: The Healing Effect of Nutritional Supplements**
Nicholas W. Read . . . 45

4.1 Why Do So Many People Feel Unwell . . . 47

4.2 The Placebo or Healing Effect 51

4.3 Who Responds to Placebo Medication 56

4.4 Nutritional Supplements as Placebos 57

4.5 The Ethics of Prescribing or Marketing Placebos as Nutritional Supplements 59

4.6 References 62

5 Antioxidants, Nutrition and Health
Anthony Diplock 65

5.1 Introduction 65

5.2 Involvement of Free Radicals in Degenerative Disease and Modulation by Antioxidants 65

5.3 Cancer Aetiology 66

5.4 Cardiovascular Disease Aetiology 68

5.5 Reduction of Disease Risk by Antioxidant Nutrients 70

5.6 Cancer 70

5.7 Cardiovascular Disease 73

5.8 References 77

6 Nutritional and Non-Nutritional Uses of Vitamin B_6
David A. Bender 81

6.1 Introduction 81

6.2 Metabolism and Metabolic Functions of Vitamin B_6 82

6.3 Requirements and Reference Nutrient Intakes 84

6.4 Potential Benefits of Higher Levels of Intake: Homocysteine Metabolism 85

6.5 Pharmacological Uses of Vitamin B_6 86
6.5.1 Side-Effects of Oral Contraceptives 88
6.5.2 Impaired Glucose Tolerance and Diabetes Mellitus 89
6.5.3 Depression 90
6.5.4 The Premenstrual Syndrome 91
6.5.5 Morning Sickness 92
6.5.6 Carpal Tunnel Syndrome 92
6.5.7 Hypertension 93

6.6 Drug Interactions with Vitamin B_6 94

6.7 Toxicity of Vitamin B_6 95

6.8 References 96

7 Folic Acid and Disease Prevention: A Long Day's Journey Into Light
Christopher Schorah 101

7.1 Introduction 101

7.2 Folate Prevention of Neural Tube Defects 101

7.3 Other Congenital Malformations and Folate 104

7.4 Folate, Homocysteine and Occlusive Vascular Disease 104

7.5 Folate Requirements and Provision 105

7.6 Changed Diet 106

7.7 Supplements 106

7.8 Food Fortification 107

7.9 Conclusions 108

7.10 References 108

8 The Addition of Micronutrients to Food
H. Frank Woods 111

8.1 Introduction 111

8.2 The Historical Background 111

8.3 Some Definitions 113

8.4 The Rationale for the Addition of Nutrients to Food 114

8.5 Policy Considerations 114

8.6 Legislative Aspects of Micronutrients Addition to Food 116

8.7 The Efficacy of the Addition of Micronutrients to Food 117

8.8 References 118

9 Probiotics and Prebiotics in Health
Colette Shortt, Seppo Salminen, and Marcel Roberfroid 119

9.1 Introduction 119

9.2 Probiotic Bacteria in Human Health: An Overview
Colette Shortt and Seppo Salminen 120

9.2.1 Introduction 120
9.2.2 Probiotics and Dietary Modulation 120
9.2.3 Concept of Probiotic Bacteria 122
9.2.4 Selection of Probiotic Strains 123
9.2.5 Conclusion 127

9.3 Prebiotics in Human Health: An Overview
Marcel Roberfroid 128
9.3.1 Introduction 128

9.3.2 The Prebiotics 128
9.3.3 Malabsorption of the Non-Digestible Oligosaccharides 130
9.3.4 Fermentation in the Large Bowel: The Prebiotic Effect 131
9.3.5 Physiological Effects in the Gastro-Intestinal Tract 132
9.3.6 Prebiotics and the Risk of Colon Cancer 133
9.3.7 Conclusion: Prebiotics, What Benefit(s) for Human Health? 134
9.3.8 Conclusions 135

9.4 References 136

10 Phytoestrogens and Health
Janet Cade, Victoria Burley, and Sara Kirk 141

10.1 Introduction 141
10.1.1 Phytoestrogens – What are They and Where do we Find Them? . 141
10.1.2 Isoflavones 142
10.1.3 Coumestans 143
10.1.4 Lignans 143

10.2 Dietary Intake 143
10.2.1 Baby Foods 144
10.2.2 Key Points 145
10.2.3 Effects on Health 146

10.3 Heart Disease 146
10.3.1 Phytoestrogens May Reduce Blood Cholesterol Levels 146
10.3.2 Other Possible Effects of Phytoestrogens on CHD Risk 147
10.3.3 Key Points 147

10.4 Cancer 147
10.4.1 General Effects of Phytoestrogens 147
10.4.2 Breast Cancer 148
10.4.3 Prostate Cancer 149
10.4.4 Other Cancers 149
10.4.5 Key Points 150

10.5 Osteoporosis 150

10.6 Key points 151

10.7 Menopausal Symptoms 151
10.7.1 Key Points 152

10.8 Potential Adverse Effects 152

10.9 Conclusions and Recommendations 153

10.10 References 153

11 Dietary Supplements and their Role in the Prevention and Treatment of Coronary Heart Disease
Peter Jackson, Lawrence Ramsay, and Erica Wallis 157

11.1 Introduction 157

11.2 Evidence 158

11.3 Early Attempts at Dietary Modification to Prevent CHD 159

11.4 The Diet Trials 160
11.4.1 Fish 161
11.4.2 Nuts 162
11.4.3 Fibre 163

11.5 Homocysteine 164

11.6 Antioxidants 165
11.6.1 Vitamin C 166
11.6.2 β-carotene 166
11.6.3 Vitamin E 167

11.7 Alcohol 169

11.8 Plant Sterols and Stanols 169

11.9 Conclusion 170

11.10 References 171

12 The Scientific Basis for Fish Oil Supplementation in Rheumatoid Arthritis
Philip Calder 175

12.1 Introduction 175

12.2 Fatty Acids in the Human Diet 175

12.3 The Immune System 180
12.3.1 What is the Immune System and How Does it Work? 180
12.3.2 Communication Within the Immune System: Cytokines 182
12.3.3 Inflammation 183
12.3.4 Integration of the Immune Response 185
12.3.5 The Immune System in Health and Disease 186

12.4 Rheumatoid Arthritis 187

12.5 Eicosanoids: The Link Between Fatty Acids and the Immune System 188
12.5.1 Eicosanoid Synthesis 188
12.5.2 Roles for Eicosanoids in Inflammation and Immunity 189
12.5.3 Eicosanoids and RA 189
12.5.4 Fish Oil and Eicosanoids 190

12.6 Effects of Fish Oil on Immune Function 190

12.7 Fish Oil Intervention in Rheumatoid Arthritis 192

12.8 Conclusions and Comments 194

12.9 References 195

Contributors

Dr. David A. Bender
Department of Biochemistry and Molecular Medicine,
University College London WC1E 6BT, UK

Dr. Victoria Burley
The Nuffield Institute for Health, University of Leeds LS2 9PL, UK

Dr. Janet Cade
The Nuffield Institute for Health, University of Leeds LS2 9PL, UK

Dr. Philip Calder
Institute of Human Nutrition, University of Southampton,
Southampton S016 7PX, UK

Professor Anthony Diplock
International Antioxidant Research Centre, Guy's,
King's College and St Thomas's Hospitals Medical and Dental School,
London SE1 9RT, UK

Dr. Judith K. Donnelly
Public Health Nutrition Unit, Trinity and All Saints,
College of the University of Leeds, Leeds LS18 5HD,UK

Dr. Peter Jackson
Section of Clinical Pharmacology and Therapeutics, University of Sheffield,
Royal Hallamshire Hospital, Sheffield S10 2JF, UK

Matthew E. Joynson
Independent Research Nutritionist, *e-mail:* matthew@joynson.com

Dr. Sara Kirk
The Nuffield Institute for Health, University of Leeds LS2 9PL, UK

Professor Lawrence Ramsay
Section of Clinical Pharmacology and Therapeutics, University of Sheffield,
Royal Hallamshire Hospital, Sheffield S10 2JF, UK

Joan K. Ransley
Public Health Nutrition Unit, Trinity and All Saints,
College of the University of Leeds, Leeds LS18 5HD, UK

Professor Nicholas W. Read
The Centre for Integrated Medicine,
Institute for General Practice and Primary Care,
University of Sheffield,
Northern General Hospital, Sheffield S5 7AU, UK

Professor Marcel Roberfroid
Université Catholique de Louvain, 1180 Brussels, Belgium

Professor Seppo Salminen
Health and Biosciences, University of Turku, 20014 Turku, Finland

Dr. Christopher Schorah
Chemical Pathology, Division of Clinical Sciences,
University of Leeds LS2 9JT, UK

Dr. Colette Shortt
Science Department, Yakult London W3 7XS, UK

Dr. Erica Wallis
Section of Clinical Pharmacology and Therapeutics, University of Sheffield,
Royal Hallamshire Hospital, Sheffield S10 2JF, UK

Professor H. Frank Woods
Division of Molecular and Genetic Medicine, University of Sheffield,
Royal Hallamshire Hospital, Sheffield S10 2JF, UK

1 The Rise and Rise of Food and Nutritional Supplements – an Overview of the Market

Joan K. Ransley

1.1 Introduction

Consumers in the UK spend between £340 and £360 million each year on vitamins, minerals and dietary supplements and they form one of the largest over the counter [OTC] healthcare sectors in the UK [1] This compares with the £550 million annual UK spend on organic foods and £11.74 billion spend on fruit and vegetables [2, 3]. Across Western Europe, the market for on vitamins, minerals and dietary supplements is growing and it increased in value by 12% between 1994 and 1998 [4]. The market for these products is highly fragmented and contains an extensive list of goods, ranging from single and multivitamin preparations to tonics, which contain mixtures of herbal preparations and micronutrients.

The purpose of this chapter is to provide an overview of this lucrative market, including an analysis of the core products, major financial players, consumer profiles and driving forces behind the growth of this market across Europe.

1.2 The Products

The market for vitamins, minerals and dietary supplements can be thought of as comprising three main sectors. Firstly, single and multivitamin preparations which may be presented as tablets, capsules, powders and liquids. Secondly, dietary supplements, which include minerals, fish oils, evening primrose oil, garlic, ginseng etc, in either tablet or capsule form, and finally tonics, which are presented in either tablet or liquid form and which tend to be a combination of herbal mixtures, supplemented with micronutrients. In addition to these three categories, functional foods have appeared as a new and vibrant sector.

Table 1 shows the most popular sector of the vitamin and supplement category is cod liver oil followed by multivitamin, and mineral products. Within these sectors, products are further stratified and branded to appeal to the needs, values and beliefs of different consumers. In recent years there has been a notable development of nutritional supplements formulated for stages and conditions related to the life cycle. The formulation of these product ranges is usually linked to the specific nutritional requirement of natural states associated with stages in the life cycle e.g. rapid growth during adolescence and pregnancy. In addition,

Table 1. Sales of vitamins minerals and dietary supplements in the UK

Sales in 1998	£ million	% share of the market
Cod liver oil [CLO] and other fish oils	94	28
Multivitamins	75	22
Single vitamins	54	16
Evening primrose oil	37	11
Minerals	24	7
Garlic	17	5
Ginseng	10	3
Tonics	6	2
Others	21	6
Total	340	100

Source: Mintel Marketing Intelligence.

there are formulations associated with the symptoms associated with menstruation, the menopause and pregnancy. e.g. breast pain, hot flushes and morning sickness. Themed supplements are also beginning to appear. A range of Mediterranean diet supplements were launched recently and contained compounds frequently found in the diet of populations inhabiting the southern Mediterranean countries. The range included extracts of red wine (flavonoids), chicory inulin (oligosacharides), 'heart health' tablets (Omega-3 fatty acids), and tomato lycopene (flavonoids). Each of these food components has been associated with physiological processes involved in reducing risk factors for coronary heart disease, cancer or gastrointestinal complaints.

Formulations designed for people with particular lifestyles are appearing in major retail outlets for nebulous states such as 'hectic lifestyles' as well as better defined dietary regimens such as vegetarianism and slimming. Supplements for cosmetic effects like nourishing skin and enhancing eye health are also readily available, and illustrate the niche approach to marketing these products.

1.3 What are People Taking?

1.3.1 Cod Liver Oil

Cod liver oil (CLO) is classed as a supplement and it constitutes the largest segment of the market, with a 26% share. Recently CLO has been combined with other ingredients, such as vitamins to enhance its nutritional profile. Patients often take fish oil supplements for inflammatory conditions such as rheumatoid arthritis. This group of supplements share many of the features of a conventional medical treatment where the biochemical mechanisms involved in the aetiology of disease are modulated by active compounds contained within the food supplement and supported by randomised controlled trials [5]. Cod liver oil is a rich source of omega-3 (also known as *n*-3) fatty acids, which as Philip

Calder explains in Chapter 12 gives rise to a group of metabolically active ingredients known as eicosanoids. These play a key role in damping down the inflammatory response, which is activated in conditions such as rheumatoid arthritis.

1.3.2 Multivitamins

Multivitamin preparations are combinations of either vitamins, or vitamins and minerals. These products are designed to take the guesswork out of selecting a supplement and accounted for 22% of the UK sales of vitamin, mineral and dietary supplements in 1998 (Table 1). Multivitamins are usually formulated to provide 100% of the Reference Nutrient Intake for key micronutrients [6]. Multivitamin preparations are often taken by people who want to use a supplement as an insurance against ill health, but who cannot readily distinguish between different micronutrients and their biochemical function in the body.

1.3.3 Single Vitamins

Sales of single vitamins account for 16% of the market share. They have in recent years been the focus of intense media interest and bad press due to a number of scares associated with their use. This has affected sales in some sectors. Bad press, in the UK, included the recent spat between the House of Commons Agriculture Select Committee and the government's Food Advisory Committee about the safety and use of vitamin B_6 which gave rise to a great deal of adverse publicity concerning the efficacy of this vitamin and the limits of its role as a medicine or therapeutic agent [7]. Scares have included the findings from the randomised trial of α-tocopherol and β-carotene supplements and their effect on increasing the incidence of major coronary events in patients with previous myocardial infarction [8] and recent adverse publicity of the effects of taking mega doses of vitamin C on arterial wall growth [9]. The adverse publicity surrounding these vitamin supplements may explain the reduced enthusiasm some consumers have for taking doses of single vitamins to ward off colds, coronary heart disease and cancer.

The Health Education folic acid awareness campaign, which ran between autumn 1995 and spring 1998, has increased awareness of the need for periconceptional supplementation with this vitamin. Almost 50% of women of childbearing age are now aware of the benefits of taking folic acid to prevent neural tube abnormalities compared with the figure of 9% in 1995 [10].

1.3.4 Evening Primrose Oil

Evening primrose oil is extracted from the seeds of the plant *Oenothera biennis* and contains linoleic acid, γ-linolenic acid and vitamin E. γ-linolenic acid is a precursor of prostaglandin E and several other biologically active substances. It is the component of evening primrose oil that has been held largely accountable for its putative therapeutic effects [11]. Evening primrose oil has been tested in controlled clinical trials for the following conditions: atopic dermatitis, rheumatoid arthritis, diabetic neuropathy, multiple sclerosis, Raynaud's phenomenon, ulcerative colitis, pre-eclampsia, the premenstrual syndrome, schizophrenia, and hyperactivity with mixed results [11]. Evening primrose oil accounts for 11% of the market share (Table 1).

1.3.5 Minerals

Consumer interest in the UK in minerals such as calcium, iron, zinc and magnesium has increased by approximately 243% between 1994 and 1998. Market research has shown this interest has stemmed from an increased awareness of the role of calcium in the aetiology of osteoporosis.

1.3.6 Garlic Products

Garlic products have long been associated with reducing risk factors for cardiovascular disease. Essential oils contained within garlic have been shown to reduce platelet aggregation and to lower plasma triacylglycerol and cholesterol concentrations [12]. The active components are thought to be ajoene formed from alline (the substance that gives garlic its characteristic smell) and an enzyme allinase, which is produced when garlic is crushed. The composition of garlic capsules does not always contain these components particularly if they are derived from steam distillates [12]. Sales of garlic supplements are in decline, mainly because the younger age group consumes garlic as a part of their regular diet. It has been estimated that 3–5 g of crushed fresh garlic per day should have clinically significant effects [12]. As Table 1 shows garlic products account for only 5% of sales.

1.3.7 Functional Foods

Functional foods have evolved as a category in their own right and are not always considered as a food supplement. Definitions of functional foods vary, but they are usually familiar foods and drinks, to which a functional component is added. The functional component has a specific physiological role in the body, which has the potential to confer a health benefit [2]. Functional foods are an important entry into this field because they have been identified as a potential competitor to the sections of the supplement market as well as the fast growing organic food market. This emerging sector was expected to grow more than £300 million in the UK by the end of the year 2000 [2]. Functional foods were first developed in Japan in the mid-1980s where a demographic shift towards an older population concerned with preventing chronic disease occurred. They capitalise on consumer and media interest in new hypotheses relating to components in foods, which effect biochemical processes in the body and may have subtle effects on the aetiology of disease. They are also popular because they often confirm aspects of existing eating habits are beneficial to health, e.g. flavonoids in red wine have a role in protecting against coronary heart disease.

The main sectors in this market are yoghurts, breakfast cereals, margarine, low fat spreads, bread, eggs and juice drinks. The additional of functional ingredients is diverse and includes:

- bread fortified with folic acid, plant oestrogens, evening primrose oil and calcium,
- eggs described as "super healthy" because they are rich in omega-3 fatty acids, folic acid, iron and calcium,
- juices enriched with 'tiger root', ginseng, hemp, echinacea, lactobacillus and other macro and micronutrients,
- yoghurts containing plant sterols and stanols, acidophilus, bifidus and thermophilus cultures,
- breakfast cereals containing folic acid and other nutrients.

Growth in the functional food market is expected to continue with line extensions, brand developments and new functional ingredients [2].

1.4 Growth Across Western Europe

Across the following five European countries, UK, Italy, Germany, Spain and France there has been an increased growth in sales of micronutrients (vitamins and minerals) and dietary supplements, between 1994–1998. This has ranged from 1.4% growth in Germany to 61% in Italy. Over the same period, growth in the UK market alone has been 55%. If this market is split into just two core categories-vitamins (including multivitamins) and dietary supplements (including mineral supplements, fish oils, tonics and others), vitamins are more popular in Italy and the UK however in France, Germany and Spain the opposite is true. In France, dietary supplements account for two thirds of the sales, probably because the French are enthusiastic purchasers of tonics, nutritive drinks and herbal products. This coupled with the relaxation of sales of vitamins in France has meant the price has been driven down and vitamins are now more available in cheaper mass-market outlets and consequently account for a smaller market share.

In Spain, calcium supplements lead the dietary supplement sector although due to the recent promotion of milk as the best source of dietary calcium, sales have suffered. In Germany 'other' dietary supplements, tonics and nutritive drinks lead this sector with cure-alls known as *Melissengeiste* leading the field.

In Italy the market for dietary supplements is underdeveloped and consumers are showing evidence of experimentation with a range of products which have become more available and perceived to be suitable for a variety of needs. Sales of multivitamins and vitamin E have been particularly strong. In the UK market growth has been attributed to growing consumer sophistication in the requirements for single vitamins and the launch of specialised multivitamin ranges.

According to market research carried out by Mintel, UK consumers perceive vitamins as a 'boost' to the system whereas dietary supplements are viewed more as remedies for dietary deficiencies [1]. Reference is made later in this chapter to whether this consumer perception of dietary deficiencies is indeed justified.

1.5 Who Manufactures Vitamin, Mineral and Dietary Supplements?

Multinational companies such as Roche, Merck, Novartis, American Home Products and SmithKline Beecham share the manufacture of vitamins and dietary supplements supplied across Europe (Table 2). There are a number of niche sectors in the market, which allow the entry of small, specialist manufacturers who can focus on supplying specialist products to different retail sectors, for example, pharmacy, health food stores, and grocery distribution [4].

1.6 Retail Distribution of Vitamins, Minerals and Dietary Supplements

Current legislation across Europe permits the sale of vitamins, minerals and dietary supplements in grocery outlets such as supermarkets, health food shops, drug stores and pharmacies. In France, Spain, Italy and the UK the bulk of sales are through pharmacies. Table 3 indicates in the UK, the proportion of sales

Table 2. Value manufacturer shares of vitamins and dietary supplements by country 1999

	% value				
	France	Germany	Italy	Spain	UK
Roche Group	7.7	–	14.6	12.2	18.1
American Home Products	–	2.7	10.2	4.3	2.7
Novartis	2.1	6.9	11.1	4.2	–
Arkopharma	17.0	–	–	–	–
Juve Santé	10.6	–	–	–	–
Boehringer Ingelheim	–	4.3	–	8.2	
Taisho Pharmaceutical	–	–	–	–	–
Otsuka Pharmaceutical	–	–	–	–	–
SmithKline Beecham	2.7	17.6	–	–	–
MCM Klosterfrau	–	13.6	–	–	–
Amway	–	–	–	–	–
Merck	–	–	–	2.1	20.2
Rexall Sundown	–	–	–	–	–
General Nutrition	–	–	–	–	–
Twinlap Corp	–	–	–	–	–
Private label	0.4	1.1	–	–	38.6
Others	59.5	53.7	64.1	69.0	20.4
Total	100.0	100.0	100.0	100.0	100.0

Source: Euromonitor Market Direction (Vitamins and Dietary Supplements – July 2000).

Table 3. UK sales of vitamins and dietary supplements by retail outlet 1998

	£ million	% share of sales
Boots	102	30
Other pharmacy chains	34	10
Grocery multiples	88	26
Health food shops	55	16
Drug stores	44	13
Others	17	5
Total	340	100

Source: Mintel Marketing Intelligence.

through pharmacies has been maintained due to the prominence of Boots The Chemist, which accounts for approximately 30% of sales in 1998 [1,4].

In the UK Boots has increased its share of sales by 22% since 1994. Boots have excellent market penetration because it has a large number of stores and a high percentage of own label products at a competitive price. However there is fierce competition in the area by grocery multiples and drug stores. Grocery multiples, which include supermarkets, have experienced an increase of 57% and drug stores have experienced an increase of 47% in the same period. Chemist shops are able to capitalise on the trusted presence of a pharmacist able to give professional advice on medical aspects of product selection. Vitamin and mineral supplements are often displayed close to the pharmacy counter which makes this possible. This serves to endorse products on sale in chemist shops and adds value to the purchase.

1.7 What is Driving the Growth in this Market?

There are four key driving forces behind the growth of this market. The first is a loss of consumer confidence in the ability of the modern diet to provide all the nutrients required to maintain health and to enjoy life. Consumers perceive food as highly processed and unable to deliver the correct balance of nutrients in the appropriate amounts required to meet the heavy demands of life in the 21st century. Nutritional supplements offer a short cut to being healthy and getting back on track to a healthy diet at a time when eating regular balanced meals is in decline. They have a powerful symbolic significance and even if supplement has no measurable biological effect in the body, the influence they have on how a person may feel is all important. This is born out by research which shows that many consumers are only occasional users of supplements and take them during times of stress, following weight reducing regimens and when the spirits are low. The second driving force in the market is the ageing population who have concerns relating to preventing arthritis, cancer, coronary heart disease and osteoporosis [1]. In this group, supplements are taken as a way of preventing or treating age related symptoms and illnesses. As the European population ages the demand for supplements is forecast to develop to meet their needs. The third driving force is a growing trend towards self-medication, which has been developing in the UK and other European countries over recent years as a response to changes in healthcare provision. Consumers are more interested than ever in buying medicines, without the inconvenience, concerns about disclosure and expense of seeing a doctor [13]. Finally, an overall increase in health awareness and disease prevention among consumers has led to a greater interest in food and nutritional supplements.

1.7.1 Age and Lifestyle Trends Spin the Market

The target group index (TGI) annual survey of 25,000 adults showed that 40.9% of consumers were users of vitamin and other supplements.

By far the greatest users of food and nutritional supplements are the older age groups – 55 years and above when age related ailments come to the fore (Table 4). Men lag behind women in their use of vitamin supplements and the profile of the regular user tends to be female and aged 45 years and above. Of the 15,000

Table 4. Use of vitamins and other supplements by sex and age

	% sample who use vitamins and supplements	% heavy users	% medium users	% light users	% non users
All	40.9	31.4	2.9	6.6	59.1
Men	35.3	25.5	3.1	6.6	64.7
Women	46.2	37	2.6	6.6	53.8
15–24 yrs	33.4	21.3	3.4	8.6	66.6
25–34 yrs	36.5	24.4	3.3	8.7	63.5
35–44 yrs	36.9	26.2	3.7	7	63.1
45–54 yrs	44.7	37.9	2.7	5.1	55.3
55–64 yrs	46.7	39	2.3	5.4	53.3
>65 yrs	47.9	41.4	1.7	4.8	52.1

Taken from TGI annual survey sample of 25,560 adults. Source: TGI, BMRB 1998/Mintel.

Table 5. Socio-economic profile of users of vitamins and other supplements

Socio-economic group	
AB	47
C1	44
C2	38
D	36
E	35

Taken from TGI annual survey sample of 25,560 adults.
Source: TGI, BMRB 1998/Mintel.

women participating in the UK Women's Cohort Study 60% reported taking dietary supplements, which were three to four times higher than the figure reported by Gregory et al. [14,15]. There is also an association between use and income, with higher socio-economic groups being the main users (Table 5). Further data from the UK Women's Cohort Study has shown that the mean annual expenditure per person was £88, although the range was wide spanning from £5 to £360. In addition those from higher socio-economic groups spent more on supplements than those from lower socio-economic groups [16].

1.7.2 The Trend Towards Self-Medication

1.7.2.1 *Concerns About Illness Drive Demand*

Concerns about health are certainly a major reason why people choose to buy supplements. According to recent research conducted by the British Market Research Bureau for Mintel, the major health concerns for UK adults were arthritis (22%) and cancer (21%) followed by risk factors for cardiovascular disease such as high blood pressure (19%), high cholesterol levels (18%). 13% of women were concerned about osteoporosis, which matched the 13% of men concerned about prostate cancer [2]. Anxiety about these conditions rises with age with 42% of over 64 year olds expressing worries about arthritis. Interestingly arthritis is of particular concern to lower socio-economics groups [2]. Worries about high blood pressure increase with age and are particularly prevalent in higher socio-economic groups who are also concerned about obesity and cholesterol levels. While blood pressure concern is associated with ageing, high cholesterol levels concerns all age groups over 24 years and higher rather than lower socio-economic groups. This concern is probably well founded given that serum cholesterol levels of the average older adult in Western countries is high (6.0–6.5 mmol/l) [17]. Concerns and anxieties about health among these demographic sub groups makes them an ideal target for functional foods such as margarines containing plant sterols and stanols such as Benecol and Flora Pro-activ, which are flagship functional products. Plant sterols and stanols reduce the absorption of cholesterol from the gut and lower serum cholesterol [18]. Sterols are an essential component of cell membranes and both animals and plants produce them. The sterol ring is common to all sterols and the difference is in the side chain. Cholesterol is exclusively an animal sterol and there are over 40 plant sterols (phytosterols) which have been identified. Stanols are less abundant in nature but they can be manufactured by hydrogenating sterols. There is good evidence to show that including 2 g of plant sterol or stanol in an average daily portion of margarine reduces serum levels of low density lipoprotein by enough to cause a 25% reduction in the risk of heart disease. It would however add an extra £70 per year to a person's food bill as each 250 g tub costs about £2.50 compared to 60p for a typical polyunsaturated margarine [18]. Needless to say there is a ready market for these products with the relatively affluent, ageing population who have concerns relating to cardiovascular disease.

Two emerging health trends have been identified recently and could influence new product development especially in the functional food market. The first relates to making the immune system function more efficiently by taking herbs such as echinacea and secondly alleviating the symptoms of mild to moderate depression using Hypericum perforatum (St John's wort).

Interest in the medicinal use of these herbs has grown both among consumers and doctors [19–21]. Health professionals and consumers are increasingly concerned about the health effects of stressful lifestyles and as a result of this products which 'calm' anxious states and aid sleep are growth areas [1, 22].

1.7.2.2
Changes in the Pharmacy

In addition over recent years an increasing number of medicines have moved from prescription – only medicines (POM), to pharmacy medicines (P) which can be bought under the supervision of a pharmacist. Also some P listed medicines have been designated to the General Sales List (GSL) where they can be purchased freely from a number of retail outlets such as supermarkets. The result in this overhaul of the classification of medicines is that patients and consumers are able to self prescribe therapies which were once only available from a GP. This increase in self-medication has increased consumer confidence and willingness to purchase food and nutritional supplements for common ailments e.g. mega doses of vitamin C for the common cold.

The soaring price of prescription medicines and increasing difficulties accessing national health service care, have lead to patients becoming more willing to take a greater degree of personal responsibility for their treatment and healthcare. In addition general practitioners recognise the need for responsible self-medication in treating common conditions. This has lead to an increase in self-medication in treating minor conditions. Whilst vitamin supplements are not medicines they have benefited from the overall growth of the 'over the counter' (OTC) healthcare market [13].

1.7.2.3
Changes in Primary Health Care

Recent changes in primary health care have resulted in an across the board increase in self-medication. These changes have lead to an alteration in the role of the pharmacist who the government has given greater powers to deal with the type of minor illnesses that clog up doctors' surgeries. Despite this there is some evidence that family doctors are advising the use of vitamins and also supplements for patients who are older, to treat age related conditions and for pre-family patients [1].

1.8 Do Supplement Users Need to Take Supplements?

It is widely reported that the nutritional intakes of users of food supplements meets current nutritional guidelines specified by the Department of Health [6, 14, 23]. Comparing the dietary intake (minus supplements) of a group of supplement users and non users, Kirk showed that supplement users had higher intakes of all nutrients except for fat and vitamin $B_{12.}$ Vegetarians, those who ate a lot of fruit and vegetables, those who drank little alcohol and who exercised regularly were all more likely to take supplements [14]. The lifestyle and nutrient intake of supplement users support the 'inverse supplement hypothesis' which states that those who do not actually need supplements are more likely to take them [24]. Data from the Women's Cohort Study provided evidence of excessive doses of certain vitamins. One respondent consumed a daily intake of 9 g of vitamin C, from vitamin C supplements and an additional 90 mg from another vitamin preparation resulting in an intake of over 200 times the RNI. This was without taking her dietary intake into account [23].

The evidence presented above suggests that consumers who take vitamin and mineral supplements do not usually need them. This leads to speculations about why they choose to take them. In part their supplement taking behaviour may be driven by their concern for optimal nutritional intake, which even experts in the nutritional field debate vigorously.

Establishing how much of a nutrient is enough without becoming too much is one of the most problematic areas that nutritionists have to address. The long term consequences of consuming too much energy are obvious as a positive energy balance can lead to weight gain. With regard to micronutrients the situation is different because deciding the optimum intake for an individual person is complex. The bioavailablity of a micronutrient varies according to the interactions between the nutrient and other nutrients and non- nutrients. It also depends on nutrient requirements such as lifestyle factors (e.g. smoking, exercise) and genetic variability which all make determining an individuals requirement uncertain [25].

When determining the requirements for nutrients, there is currently more emphasis placed on considering the kinds of nutrients needed to optimise physiological and mental functions and to minimise the development of degenerative diseases, rather than simply preventing deficiency states. This approach recognises that nutrient activity may take place at a multiplicity of levels as follows:

1. the amount of a nutrient which may prevent an overt nutritional disease
2. the amount of a nutrient which may optimise biochemical, physiological and genetic functions associated with specific health benefits
3. the pharmacological dose of a nutrient needed to optimise non-traditional functions associated with specific health benefits
4. the amount of a nutrient which may lead to specific health hazards or toxic effects.

Current dietary recommendations are based on the concept of 'essentiality', which refers to the amount of a nutrient required to prevent disease. The amounts are determined by observational and experimental findings. A less rigid definition of essentiality would embrace the notion of 'optimum' nutrition and would involve considering a dietary factor a 'nutrient' if it affects the metabolism of a person in a way that is beneficial to health. Revising the concept of essentiality to determine and recognise the multiple levels of nutrient action is currently being explored [25].

The notion of optimum nutrition is attractive to consumers who doubt both the ability of their diet to provide the nutrients required to prevent nutrient deficiencies and to deliver the optimum range and level of nutrients to maximise their health and prevent disease. Given that there is no consensus among nutritionists about optimum requirements for some nutrients or dietary components it is hardly surprising that some consumers take the issue into their own hands. Levels of intake can be based on unverified sources of advice such as health food shops, the media and complementary therapists. This approach to self-medication carries risks and there is evidence that intakes of some supplements can be deleterious to health and lead to acute adverse effects such as diarrhoea (vitamin C) and flushing (niacin). Persistent more serious adverse effects are rare for water soluble vitamins although chronic use of high doses of vitamin B_6 can lead to neuropathies. High doses of fat soluble vitamins are of greater concern: vitamin A has been linked to birth defects and irreversible bone and liver damage and vitamin D with hypercalcaemia. High does of single minerals or amino acids may induce deficiency in nutrients which share similar nutritional pathways. Excessive doses of zinc and selenium can cause immune suppression and evening primrose oil may exacerbate temporal lobe epilepsy [5].

1.9 Regulating the Market

Vitamins, minerals and dietary supplements are classified as foods and regulated by the 1990 Food Safety Act. The claims that are made for the use and efficacy of such products are regulated by the Food Labelling Regulations 1996. Medicines are regulated by separate legislation laid out in the Medicines Act or the Medicines for Human Use Regulations 1994. The claims which can be made about a medicine are different from those that can be made about a dietary supplement. In the UK most vitamins, minerals and dietary supplements are regulated as foods and they may be freely sold in supermarkets, health food shops and pharmacies. This means that dietary supplements may not be promoted for medicinal use, or make any claim that a product can prevent or cure specific illnesses. However food and pharmaceutical industries can make health promoting claims such as 'this product helps to lower cholesterol', provided the claim can be substantiated by sound science and is not misleading [2]. Claims made about supplements cannot assert disease treatment or prevention [26]. The regulation of food supplements across Europe varies and there is pressure from the EU Commission in Brussels to harmonise legislation across the European Union. Recently the EU Commission proposed new legislation that would required a number of changes to be put in place. For example, labels on the packaging of vitamin supplements will be required to include a recommendation for a daily dose, a warning about possible health risks associated with high intakes and a message stating that the product should not be used as a substitute for a varied diet. Packaging will also be required to clearly identify the difference between a food supplement and a medicinal product. There are also plans to include a positive list of vitamins, minerals and chemical substances that have been approved as safe by the EU's food scientific committee. If EU governments and the European parliament agree with the proposals, they could become law in 2002 and any products not complying with its terms would have to be taken off the market [27].

The Joint Health Claims Initiative (JHCI) has been instigated recently by a partnership between the food industry, the regulators LACOTS (Local Authority co-ordinating Body on Food and Trading Standards) and consumer interests, and will provide a framework for harmonising the processes used to assess claims in the UK. The Code Administration Body for the JHCI is expected to be situated within Leatherhead Food RA. If the JHCI is adopted throughout the food and supplements industry it should hopefully protect the public against misleading marketing activities [28].

Recent developments in the USA regulations have in effect relaxed the tight restrictions governing the claims made for the health benefits of herbal supplements and may further influence legislation in Europe [29]. The decision made by the US Food and Drug Administration (FDA) has opened the way for manufacturers of vitamins, herbs and dietary supplements to manufacture products for conditions such as morning sickness, hot flushes and memory loss in ageing. The significant feature of the new law states that manufacturers of dietary supplements can make claims about how their products affect the structure and function of the body. They may not, however, claim to prevent, treat, cure, mitigate or diagnose a disease without FDA approval. The new law is part of the Dietary Supplement Health and Education Act. This act allows manufacturers to sell products without the FDA's rigorous safety and efficacy review which is required for drugs, as long as they make claims related only to how a product affects the 'structure or function of the body' and not how they affect disease states.

Despite the existing regulations many consumers and patients have high expectations about the role of dietary supplements in the prevention, treatment and cure of disease. In part this is due to the way the media sensationalises new research findings and promotes the use of supplements in articles appearing in lifestyle publications such as women's magazines and Sunday newspapers. The industry does however rely on media reports to sell its products. With a limited scope for advertising copy, manufacturers are hidebound by the regulations governing what they may claim. A well written article in an influential newspaper however has a lot more freedom to provide the indirect sales push for a product or product category. It is well known in the industry that a strong recommendation from women's magazine such as Good Housekeeping is all that is needed for sales of a product to soar [1]. Health food shops rely also on 'in house' magazines to feature articles on the health benefits of supplements thus giving more leeway for claims and suggestions which cannot be made by law on packaging and in advertising. Media reports can also work against the interests of manufacturers and retailers of supplements by running sensational scare stories for example 'Warning from scientists over high doses of dietary supplements [9].

1.10 The Future for Vitamins, Minerals and Dietary Supplements

Across Western Europe the growth in the market for vitamins, minerals and dietary supplements is set to continue. Euromonitor predicts a value increase of 21% between 1998 and 2003. The Italian market is forecast to grow by 64% between 1998 and 2003. This will be mainly due to the lifting of an advertising ban on these products. The UK market is also forecast to grow by 41% over the same period whilst the value of the market in Germany is expected to decline by about 10% [4].

The key trends that will drive this growth will be further development of self-medication. Governments are likely to switch more products from prescription only to OTC or general sales list status as a way of reducing the burden of healthcare costs on public spending. This will support the expansion of the OTC sector and benefit sales of vitamins, minerals and dietary supplements which are forecast to become the second most popular type of OTC healthcare after analgesics [13]. The market will also benefit from the expansion of the ageing population across Western Europe who will be willing to take dietary supplements to maintain their health. Recent figures from the Office of National Statistics show that there will be a 13% increase in the number of 55–64 year old in the UK between 2000 and 2004, which compares with an increase of 5.6% in the 6 years before the year 2000. In addition projections for the socio-economic structure of the population show an increase of 7% in the number of ABs and 4% in the C1 s. This is a major target group for vitamins, minerals, dietary supplements and functional foods.

As products become more mainstream, retail distribution will move away from pharmacies and into grocery outlets and health food shops. This will encourage the further development of private labelled products, particularly in the grocery sector. Consumers are expected to become more sophisticated in their choice of products which will encourage the development of more specialised products targeted at particular groups. Dietary supplements will benefit from growing health awareness of the Western European population, interest in preventative measures and growing stress at work and home. Snacking and ad hoc eating patterns are set to continue across Western Europe, with further erosion of traditional meals and the development of quick meal solutions for eating in the car and at work [30]. The growth in the market for vitamins, minerals and dietary supplements will be supported by strong promotional campaigns from manufacturers, to accompany the launch of increasingly sophisticated and specialised products targeted at niche groups.

1.11 Conclusion

Large numbers of consumers and patients are taking vitamins, minerals and dietary supplements on a daily basis. They are characteristically female, middle aged and concerned about symptoms of age related conditions such as arthritis, obesity, high blood pressure, high blood cholesterol levels and cancer. Over the next few years this trend is set to continue and with an ageing Western European population providing a larger market for these products. In addition younger people take supplements as a 'boost to their system' in times of stress and when they are feeling run down and fatigued. Niche products will proliferate to cater for an increasingly sophisticated consumer with specialist needs. Sales will become less regulated with more supplements being sold outside pharmacies and in retail outlets like supermarkets and over the Internet Media interest will continue to feast on new hypotheses and scientific findings, which support or refute the role of supplements in health and disease. As the OTC health care market grows so too will the practice of self-medication and the demand for supplements. Regulation will continue to be an issue although it is clear that most micronutrients and dietary supplements will be regulated as foods rather than medicines. The future for the industry looks bright but for the consumer and vulnerable ill patient it looks daunting as more and more products are introduced onto the market at premium prices. Consumers and patients will require help with evaluating the scientific evidence supporting the use of these products in optimising the health and preventing disease. Health professionals will need to play an important role in this regard. They will need to be alert to the needs of their patients and the reasons why they are taking these products. They will also need to be able to evaluate their biological and psychological value to the patient and to have an informed dialogue with them regarding their use. The use of vitamin, mineral and dietary supplements will also need to be evaluated in terms of the many other dietary and lifestyle changes which Western Europeans could make to improve their health and reduce risk factors for disease.

1.12 References

1. Mintel Marketing Intelligence. *Vitamins, minerals and dietary supplements.* London: Mintel International Group Ltd, 1999
2. Mintel Marketing Intelligence. *Functional foods.* London: Mintel International Group Ltd, 2000
3. Keynote. *Market review 1999, UK food market.* Middlesex, England, Keynote Ltd, 1999
4. Euromonitor. *Vitamins and dietary supplements. Market research Europe [Jan-March].* London, Euromonitor Plc, 1999
5. Vickers A, Zollman C. ABC of complementary medicine. Unconventional approaches to nutritional medicine. *BMJ* 1999; 319: 1419–1422
6. Department of Health. Dietary reference values for food energy and nutrients for the United Kingdom. London: HMSO, 1991
7. Collier J. Vitamin B-6: food or medicine? The rules-and the politics-are different. British Medical Journal 1998; 317: 92–93

8. Rapola JM, Virtamo J, Ripatti S et al. Randomised trial of α-tocopherol and β-carotene supplements on incidence of major coronary events in men with previous myocardial infarction. *Lancet* 1997; 349: 1715–1720
9. Rawstorne T. Warning from scientists over high doses of dietary supplements. Daily Mail, April 13, 2000
10. Rezan AK, Sabin C, Whitlow B, Brockbank E, Economides D. Neural tube defects and periconceptional folic acid in England and Wales: retrospective study. British Medical Journal 1999; 319: 92–93
11. Kleijnen J. Evening primrose oil. *BMJ* 1994; 309: 824–825
12. Linder M. Nutritional biochemistry and metabolism. 2nd ed. London: Prentice Hall International, 1991
13. Euromonitor. European markets OTC healthcare. London: Euromonitor Plc, 1999
14. Kirk SFL, Cade JE, Barrett JH, Conner M. Diet and lifestyle characteristics associated with supplement use in women. *Public Health Nutrition* 1999; 2: 69–73
15. Gregory J, Foster K, Tyler H, Wiseman M. The dietary and nutritional survey of British adults. London: HMSO, 1990
16. Greenhalgh A, Cade JE, Richardson C. Dietary supplement use in women-costs and frequency of use. Proceedings of the Nutrition Society. In press
17. Colhoun H, Prescott-Clarke P (eds) Health survey for England 1994. London, HMSO, 1996
18. Law M. Plant sterol and stanol margarines and health. *BMJ* 2000; 320: 861–864
19. Linde K, Ramirez G, Mulrow CD, Pauls A, Weidenhammer W, Melchart D. St John's wort for depression-an overview and meta-analsysis of randomised clinical trials. *BMJ* 1996; 313: 253–258
20. Melchart D, Linde K, Fischer P, Kaesmayr J. Echinacea for preventing and treating the common cold. In: Cochrane Collaboration. The Cochrane Library. Issue 3. Oxford: Update Software 1999
21. Vickers A, Zollman C. ABC of Complementary Medicine. Herbal medicine. *BMJ* 1999; 319: 1050–1053
22. von Onciul J. ABC of work related disorders: stress at work. *BMJ* 1996; 313: 745–748
23. Kirk SFL, Cade JE, Conner MT, Barrett JH. Supplementary issues for women. Nutrition Bulletin, 1998; 23: 197–202
24. Kirk S, Woodhouse A, Conner M. Beliefs, attitudes and behaviour in relation to supplement use in the UK Women's Cohort Study. Proceedings of the Nutrition Society, 1998 57[1], 54 A
25. Strain JJ. Optimal nutrition: an overview. Proceedings of the Nutrition Society, 1998; 58: 395–396
26. Mason P. Nutrition and dietary advice in the pharmacy. Oxford: Blackwell Scientific, 1994
27. Watson R. EU to tighten rules on dietary supplements. *BMJ* 2000; 320: 1362–1363
28. Buttriss J. Is Britain ready for FOSHU? Nutrition Bulletin, 2000; 25[2], 159–161
29. Gottlieb S. US relaxes its guidelines on herbal supplements. *BMJ* 2000; 320: 208–209
30. Euromonitor. Savoury snacks. Market Research Europe. London: Euromonitor Plc, 1999

2 Why do Health Professionals Need to Know More About Nutrition?

Matthew E. Joynson

2.1 Introduction

Nutrition and diet are fundamental to health with diet regarded as the most important environmental factor determining longevity. Although Hippocrates recognised the importance of a good diet for the prevention of disease, the science of nutrition has only emerged recently as an important discipline in modern medicine. Clearly nutrition is not just a simple case of ensuring regular consumption of the recommended daily doses of vitamins and minerals. Instead, nutritional science broadly encompasses the intake, absorption and metabolism of dietary constituents, along with the promotion of health via prevention of diet-related diseases. As we enter the 21st Century, scientific advances on the relationship of dietary substances to the cellular mechanisms of disease are occurring with increasing regularity and frequency. Yet despite the increasing scientific evidence, present day health professionals are typically untrained in the impact of diet in health and disease [1]. Furthermore, simple dietary deficiencies still occur within developed societies [2].

The array of foods and dietary supplements available to the general public continues to increase. With the advent of functional foods such as prebiotics and probiotics, and supplements containing phytochemicals, health professionals may require further scientific knowledge to offer nutritional advice to patients and consumers.

The aim of this chapter is to consider why health professionals such as dentists, pharmacists and general practitioners, need to know more about nutrition. Although the chapter offers a UK perspective on dietary knowledge in primary care, the principles and issues discussed in this chapter should equally apply to other countries.

2.1.1 The Implication of Diet in Disease

Dietary factors are influential in the most important public health problems of Western society. Diseases such as coronary heart disease, stroke, cancers and osteoporosis constitute the most common causes of morbidity and mortality [1, 3, 4]. When considering the management of diseases associated with the modern lifestyle, nutrition should be considered a primary issue. Although all of these diseases are multifactorial in their aetiology, the potential exists for disease prevention via manipulation of the diet. Diet has been estimated to a contributory factor in up to 80% of cancers of the large bowel, breast, and prostate [8, 9] – however, the direct effects of the diet are less certain, but fats, fibre and antioxidants have been closely scrutinised [7]. For coronary heart disease and stroke, dietary factors play important roles in modulating blood lipids and their propensity for oxidation [8]; diet has been linked with development of coronary atherosclerosis from an early age [9]. In addition, thrombosis can be influenced by dietary factors, particularly fish oils [10]. In osteoporosis the most important dietary factor appears to be the availability of calcium [11] which is essential both in building peak bone mass and in minimising bone loss in later life. However, therapeutic manipulation of the diet, by the addition of fish oils to increase the supply of omega-3 fatty acids to reduce the inflammatory response in rheumatoid arthritis [12] is regarded as unconventional by many health professionals.

One clear conclusion from existing epidemiologic evidence is that many individuals have suboptimal diets and that the potential for disease prevention via improved nutrition is substantial [4]. With an increased focus on individual components of the diet, the physiological and biochemical roles of these nutrients in health and disease are becoming more clearly defined. For example, low levels of plasma folate has been linked to the aetiology of cardiovascular disease [13–15]. Nutritional studies in patients with cardiovascular disease and controls have shown an inverse correlation between concentrations of vitamin B_{12} and folate and those of homocysteine. Thus, supplementation with folate in deficient patients can normalise homocysteine levels and potentially reduce the risk of cardiovascular disease [14, 15].

The provision of dietary advice is already common in the management of many chronic diseases, like hypertension and hyperlipidaemia, where over 90% of patients are exclusively managed in family medicine [16]. However the provision of dietary advice needs to extend beyond diseased patients and play a higher role in relation to healthy patients and the potential for disease prevention. As nutrition knowledge changes with new scientific evidence, the health professional must ensure that individuals are aware of the protective factor that an appropriate diet can convey to them. This health strategy may aid in preventing further morbidity and mortality.

2.2 Our Hunger for Knowledge

Nutrition is becoming increasingly important for a number of reasons. In many societies, busy lifestyles, irregular working patterns and active social lives often lead to missed meals and over indulgence in fast or convenience foods. These refined foods easily fit into modern lives but propel the trend to spend less time preparing food. However, the consumption of such foods can contribute to an insufficient diet characterised by low micronutrient density and an excess of fat. Also, many individuals are turning to alternative diets in accordance with their personal beliefs: vegetarian, vegan, and macrobiotic diets are increasingly being followed. However, many of these diets, such as veganism or macrobiotics, can be highly restrictive and associated with complications such as reduced bone mass or anaemia. With the realisation that dietary behaviour is insufficient, many individuals consider the consumption of food supplements to avoid dietary deficiency and increase daily intake of 'protective' nutrients. But what is the source of the general public's dietary knowledge?

Although government campaigns may advise the general public against smoking and drinking, limited nutrition guidance exists. In the absence of reliable medical advice on nutrition, patients are increasingly turning to the media to find out about healthy diets. Unfortunately, many consumers find themselves faced with the commercial aspect of nutrition. Dietary supplements constitute a major commercial enterprise with vast numbers of companies purporting that their nutrition supplements are the 'best', the 'most potent', or the 'cheapest'. Whilst all these factors may be important to the consumer, the frequent absence of clear nutritional advice may confuse the consumer. Vast numbers of people are turning to a diverse and sometimes bizarre array of nutrition and herbal dietary supplements offering occasionally unresearched, biochemically implausible interventions which are popularised by spectacular claims in the lay press; these dietary interventions are largely unsubstantiated and administered without professional supervision. This is a cause for concern, particularly with surveys reporting that the general public's knowledge of sources of fat, calcium, and iron is often unreliable [17]. Clearly there is a knowledge gap that needs to be filled.

Dietary messages have also become more complex over the past decade, changing from the simple directives of previous decades (for example, RDAs, etc) as scientific evidence has evolved. Evidently, the general public has become more knowledgeable, but also more confused. The constraints imposed by various media (print, radio, and television) that deliver the 'healthy diet' message may add a further layer of complexity, particularly if this message is part of a strong marketing strategy [18].

With an ever-increasing percentage of the population using the Internet as a source of dietary knowledge, the added concern exists that nutrition information may be inaccurate, inappropriate or commercially biased. Unfortunately, because of the lack of regulation, the quality of dietary information on the Internet is determined solely by the organisations and individuals that publish it. Davison [19] recently evaluated the accuracy of nutrition resources on the Internet and reported that 45% of websites visited provided information that was inaccurate with many being commercially orientated. Clearly, the need for an authoritative and respected source of dietary information exists.

2.3 Health Professionals: the Authorative Source of Nutrition Information?

A mismatch appears to exist between the attitude of the public, who appear willing to accept dietary advice from primary care professionals, and the reluctance of these professionals to fulfil this role [20]. Primary care should be seen as the ideal interface to provide nutrition education, with appropriate and accurate dietary advice communicated from any health professional in a clear and consistent manner. Pharmacists, family doctors, dentists and nurses should all be perceived as an approachable and informative source of general health information, along with the dietitian, the dedicated health professional in the area of nutrition. However, current dietary knowledge of the primary care team needs to be regularly updated in response to the population's new awareness of healthy eating benefits.

In Western societies, family medicine forms the front line of the health service and in the United Kingdom the contact rate between the population and primary care doctors now averages five encounters a year and relationships last an average of eleven years [16]. This gives primary care, particularly in the form of multiprofessional teams of doctors and nurses, a potential opportunity to explain the principles of healthy eating. All health professionals should play an active role in the dietary health of the general public, monitoring their eating behaviour and the impact of food across all social groups, with the irregularity of patient-health professional interaction heightening the importance of distinct dietary advice.

Primary health care staff are increasingly involved in the provision of dietary advice for health promotion, often without adequate training in nutrition assessment or counselling. Because of their perceived high status and contact with the community, the expertise of the primary care team can penetrate nearly all segments of the population placing physicians and pharmacists in a unique position to influence nutritional health. Their role should not focus upon curative care alone, but also disease prevention and health promotion. However, a general practitioner or nurse may not have the time to give dietary advice during the majority of consultations. This suggests that the community pharmacist or dentist could be effectively positioned within the primary care team to offer dietary advice to patients and consumers.

A patient's interaction with the pharmacist in the setting of a commercial pharmacy is more frequent than with any other member of the primary care team. Whereas the majority of health professionals tend to operate on an appointment only basis, the community pharmacist's advice is immediately available. Pharmacists are in the ideal position to offer advice on potential nutrient-drug interactions, particularly when dietary supplements share the same shelves as over-the-counter medications. The location and accessibility of community pharmacists for immediate consultation places them in a unique position and as respected health professionals, pharmacists are required to be a competent and knowledgeable source of reliable information. However, with the boom of nutrition supplements and the widely differing needs of individuals, the pharmacist needs to be aware of any relevant supportive or detrimental evidence from the scientific literature.

Similarly, dentists are in the ideal position to identify early signs of undernutrition, high sugar consumption, or potential dietary problems due to poor tooth development, oral disease, or tooth loss [21]. Thus the promotion of oral health should coincide with dietary advice.

Although the general public should perceive health professionals to be a source of accurate dietary information, a recent study reported that only 53% of individuals questioned thought that their general practitioner was a good source of dietary advice [17]. When general practitioners and nurses were questioned, a lack of confidence was apparent concerning the meaning of several nutritional terms, including extrinsic sugars, non-starch polysaccharide and *trans* fatty acids. Furthermore, although general practitioners were confident they could explain the link between diet and heart disease, they were not sure about the value of starch in the diet.

The challenge of dealing with food and nutrition misinformation is long-standing and persistent [22]. Cooperation between health professionals may help to expose emerging dietary misinformation and misbeliefs before they become widely accepted. In the past, nutrition communications have frequently placed priority on reducing fat consumption. This has served to foster an obsession with and confusion about dietary fat and has contributed to misperceptions about healthy eating [23]. Nutrition communicators are encouraged to work together to restore reason to nutrition messages and recommendations in an effort to help consumers achieve nutrition and health goals.

2.4 Nutrition: the Orphan Discipline

If health promotion in primary care is to work effectively, the infrastructure necessary for effective training and continuing education has to be addressed, particularly as health professionals worldwide are increasingly advising on lifestyle.

Nutrition education for health professionals appears to be an 'orphan' discipline with minimal improvement over the past decade. Curing rather than preventing disease appears to emphasised during training, particularly in schools of medicine and pharmacy. The nutrition education of health professionals should feature nutritional matters and encourage students to integrate knowledge gained from disciplines that they previously felt were perhaps unrelated. But is this achieved?

Considering the undergraduate training of the pharmacist, the curriculum does not appear to focus on nutrition as a separate entity – nutrition usually becomes fragmented into the subject areas of physiology, clinical pharmacy and pharmacy practice (M.E. Joynson, unpublished work). Thus, pharmacists may find themselves in a very uncomfortable and insecure position when answering the public's general nutritional queries.

On the average pharmacy shelf, nutritional supplements are commonplace suggesting that pharmacists themselves are well-qualified to give dietary advice to members of the public who enquire about diet and supplementation. However, when pharmacists are asked about dietary supplements, many cite the manufacturers recommended guidelines to be the limit of their knowledge. Upon closer examination, many pharmacy degree courses in the United Kingdom fail to offer students any significant education in the implications of diet and disease with many courses unable to incorporate core nutrition. Some educational institutions are beginning to recognise this important discrepancy: in 1990, the University of Brighton introduced an optional nutrition module into the third year of the pharmacy degree which was a 'first' for the Schools of Pharmacy in the United Kingdom. The content of this module is aimed at topical issues with which the community pharmacist may be involved and provides the opportunity to think generally about the communication of complex nutritional issues to the general public. Schools of pharmacy clearly have a duty to educate their students more thoroughly on the importance of diet.

Despite the prevalence of nutritional disorders in medicine and the increased significance of disease prevention via dietary modification, health professionals are typically untrained in the relationship of diet and its potential to prevent disease. The lack of importance attached to nutrition and prevention of disease is understandable particularly with the contrast between the often immediate efficacy of pharmacotherapy compared with more long-term dietary intervention remaining so distinctive. Furthermore, rigorous regulations for drugs to become licensed ensure that information is authoritative, evidence-based via clinical trials, and readily available in the medical literature. Nutrition information, however, still comes in a plethora of different forms, some of it unscientific, some out-of-date, and some commercially biased. Exceptions do exist, with dietary intervention such as the administration of fish oil supplements in patients with rheumatoid arthritis possessing features of a conventional medical treatment: a confirmed biochemical mechanism and supportive therapeutic evidence from randomised studies [12]. However, usage of such dietary supplementation is still considered unconventional and remains indistinguishable from less proven dietary intervention.

A recent study reported that nutrition ought to have an established place in the vocational training of general practitioners. When general practitioners were recently surveyed, 89.6% of responders agreed that nutrition had an important role to play in the management of disease [24]. Similarly, it is generally accepted that knowledge of nutrition is a fundamental aspect of professional nursing practice, yet there is increasing concern about ignorance of nutrition-related areas among practising nurses. Numerous reports have identified a serious problem of unrecognised malnutrition in UK hospitals which has significant clinical and financial consequences [25]. A lack of knowledge and understanding, attributed to inadequate nutrition education and training have been blamed as the principle reason for lack of progress in tackling the problem [26]. A recent study investigated the role of nurses and their attitudes to nutrition education and relationships with dietitians [27]. Nutrition education received during their nurse training was perceived to be poor by 38% of respondents and 44% of the respondents said that a state-registered dietitian had not been involved in their nutrition education. Overall, the lack of nutrition knowledge of health professionals appears to be a frequently reported problem.

2.5 What are the Obstacles to Giving Nutrition Advice?

Although the expanding role of health professionals has led to more opportunities to offer dietary advice to patients, obstacles appear to prevent communication of dietary information to the general public. Previous surveys have shown that there is a disparity between physicians' beliefs about the importance of diet and nutrition in health maintenance and disease prevention and the actual delivery of nutrition counselling [28]. Although two-thirds of physicians provided dietary counselling to less than 40% of patients, with on average less than five minutes spent discussing diet per consultation, nearly 75% of physicians felt that dietary counselling was both important and the responsibility of the physician.

Dissatisfaction with the quality of nutrition education received by those working in primary care is often cited as a barrier to providing dietary advice to patients [20]. A number of other perceived barriers to the delivery of dietary counselling have been examined and a number of obstacles identified. These include: lack of time, patient noncompliance, inadequate teaching materials, lack of knowledge, inadequate reimbursement, and low physician confidence [28]. Hence, the existence of multiple barriers appears to prevent the primary care practitioner from providing effective dietary counselling. Similarly, Helman [29] identified these obstacles as lack of time, lack of confidence, and inadequate nutrition knowledge which have since been confirmed [30]. However, research has indicated that further nutrition education or training can make a significant impact. Cadman and Findlay [30] assessed the changes in the nutrition knowledge and confidence of nurses following training from a dietitian. Nutrition knowledge increased after training with 88% of nurses reporting good or excellent confidence compared with 27% before training. This suggests that health professionals would benefit from further training and an update of their nutrition knowledge. Current nutrition principles and research can support the role of health professionals in providing accurate and consistent dietary advice to patients.

The prospect that health professionals will accept nutrition as an essential discipline may be enhanced by the realisation that cost-effective practice, particularly for general practitioners, can be optimised through the application of current nutrition interventions to health maintenance and patient care. The standardisation of curricula for nutrition education of health professionals would clearly contribute to the cost-effective integration of nutritional concepts into medical practice, and a multifaceted approach is required to change physician-counselling behaviour and overcome potential obstacles.

2.6 The Updated Role of Health Professionals: a New Approach

2.6.1 Tailored Dietary Advice

To enable the general public to achieve healthy objectives, health professionals must develop effective dietary interventions that address psychosocial and behavioural components of change [31]. The practice of offering more personalised dietary advice could be important. Campbell and co-workers [31] investigated two interventions in patients from family practices. The first intervention consisted of individually computer-tailored nutrition messages; the second consisted of non-tailored nutrition information based on the 1990

Dietary Guidelines for Americans with patients followed up after 4 months. The tailored intervention produced a 23% decrease of total fat intake compared with a 9% decrease in the non-tailored group. Seventy-three percent of the tailored intervention group recalled receiving a message, compared with 33% of the non-tailored intervention group. Tailored nutrition messages could be an effective tool in promoting dietary fat reduction for disease prevention or other dietary intervention.

Similarly, a recent pilot study was carried out in a community pharmacy utilising interactive public health software called Cardio*Pharm* [32]. The program gave advice on reducing the risks of cardiovascular disease and required the user to input various details of their lifestyle, with particular attention to diet, to allow any advice given to be more individual-specific. A brief risk assessment was then provided and the user was encouraged to consult health promotion leaflets provided. From the users, 71% agreed or strongly agreed that the experience made them think more clearly about their lifestyle.

2.6.2 Different People, Different Dietary Needs

Although comprehensive advice can be given to the general public, specific populations and communities have to be considered with thought given to lifestyle, location, culture and age. For example, communities in rural areas are often in receipt of general health education messages, although these messages are invariably composed without regard to where people reside, and, in particular, to the availability of, and access to, foodstuffs [33]. Similarly, although nutrition and ageing are inseparably connected (as eating patterns affect the progress of many degenerative diseases associated with ageing), there is an apparent lack of specific dietary advice given to elderly individuals. Old people living alone are particularly vulnerable to a poor diet, although they are also at risk in hospitals and residential homes, where a lack of resources and staff time means that they do not always receive a balanced diet. Malnutrition can lead to lower physical strength, greater inactivity, increased risk of accidents, and Chandra [34] has suggested an increased risk of infection. Poor vision, macular degeneration and cataracts are all now being linked to diets low in antioxidants consumed by the elderly [35]. Folate status has also been reported to be low in a significant proportion of elderly individuals, but effective dietary intervention can resolve this situation. When the diets of elderly individuals were supplemented with folate 100–200 mg/day, a 73% reduction in the risk of angina and myocardial infarction has been reported, with an average increase of eight years in lifespan [36]. Health promotion and disease prevention could improve the quality of elderly life, reduce morbidity and lessen the burden on the health care system, and as such it would seem reasonable that such efforts would be of benefit.

Other groups that need extra dietary guidance include children, athletes, people with active lifestyles, ethnic groups, individuals with limited diets (vegetarian, vegan, macrobiotics) and pregnant women. Every person has individual dietary needs and it is the responsibility of health professionals to take these needs into consideration when offering nutrition advice. However, health professionals should convey the value of a well balanced diet to any individual seeking dietary advice.

2.6.3 Drug-Nutrient Interactions

The potential interaction between drugs and nutrients is an important issue, particular in patients with chronic or comorbid conditions that may require prolonged or multiple treatment (arthritis, diabetes, psychiatric illness). To evaluate the attitudes of healthcare providers on drug-nutrient interaction counselling, a survey was sent to 100 pharmacists, 50 registered dietitians, 25 registered nurses and 25 physicians [37]. The variables assessed included the amount of drug-nutrient interaction counselling provided along with whom was thought to be in the best position to provide it. Only 12% of health professionals provided drug-nutrient interaction counselling in more than 50% of patient consultations. A large proportion (72%) of responders felt pharmacists were in the best position to discuss drug-nutrient interaction, with patients. In a more recent study, most general practitioners reported that they had little or no formal training in drug-nutrient interactions in medical school (83%) although 79% believed it was the physician's responsibility to inform patients about drug-nutrient interactions, and many thought pharmacists shared this responsibility [38].

Physicians' knowledge of drug-nutrient interactions may be improved by including nutrition education in the topics taught to physicians, nutritionists and pharmacists using several educational strategies. Nutrition educators in particular can play a role in curriculum development through the development and evaluation of materials and educational tools [38].

2.6.4 The Impact of Diet in Health Economics

The diet of the population can have a significant impact on the health economics of the nation. Taking bone health as an important nutrition-related issue, it has a major impact on health, quality of life and mortality. Osteoporosis is currently a major public health problem and with predicted demographic changes, its future health and economic impact is likely to be phenomenal. More than one-third of women, and approximately one-sixth of men, will sustain an osteoporotic fracture in their lifetime [39]. The National Health Service spends over £940 million annually treating at least 200,000 fractures, many in the elderly and all major osteoporotic fractures are associated with increased mortality [40]. Internationally, more than 1.5 million osteoporotic-related fractures occur annually, and this number is projected to increase 4-fold by the year 2050 [41]. Calcium intake in Britain appears variable and the bioavailability of calcium varies with 10–60% of that ingested actually being absorbed [42]. In 1994 results from a MAFF study indicated that less than one-third of 16–18-year-old girls (29%) consumed a diet that met the reference nutrient intake for calcium [43].

Increased calcium intake via food or supplementation can have beneficial effects on bone mass which could reduce the risk of developing osteoporosis or rate of onset. These effects would clearly have an impact on medical costs associated with osteoporosis. Calcium or dairy intervention studies have also demonstrated positive effects on bone mass in adolescent girls [44–47]. Similarly, in a review of more than twenty prospective studies, calcium supplementation prevented bone loss in postmenopausal women [48]. Calcium supplementation also appears to provide benefits with hormone replacement therapy: high calcium intake (over 1200 mg daily) increases the beneficial effect of the oestrogen on bone mass [47].

Following similar ideology, dietary interventions that may reduce the risk of cancer are of great importance, particularly as the figure for new cancer patients diagnosed each year has been estimated to rise from 10 million to 20 million by the year 2020 [50].

2.7 Conclusion

Health professionals, the body of authority that the general public consults for information on health, appear to be insufficiently informed about the role of diet in the prevention and treatment of disease. The expectation of nutrition guidance from health professionals needs to be acknowledged throughout the primary care team and steps need to be implemented to achieve this required level of knowledge. New efforts to train health professionals would be welcome, particularly in the interaction of nutrition and preventative medicine with the goal that a confident nutrition approach from health professionals will convey increased motivation and committment to improving nutrition behaviour in patients.

Health professionals have expressed an interest in learning more about nutrition, but there is still the lack of coherent, specifically-tailored teaching on the subject. The incorporation of nutrition education into the curricula of medical and pharmacy schools should be developed, increased and updated regularly with emphasis on health promotion and disease prevention. Opportunities and tools for physicians and pharmacists to become more actively involved in nutrition guidance of patients also need to be developed. To improve the training of health professionals in nutrition, universities could play a valuable role in developing relevant undergraduate courses which devote more time and attention both to knowledge about foods and nutrition and training on how to give well informed nutritional advice.

The recognition and importance of nutrition concepts will allow health professionals to implement practical aspects of health promotion and disease prevention in their patients, improve the overall health of their patients, and reduce the prevalence of global disease. The important and potentially cost-effective roles for the health professional in the prevention of diet-related disease are the sourcing, objective assessment and reinforcement of nutrition information. Obstacles to nutrition counselling also need to be identified and resolved.

In modern society, following an appropriate diet and a judicious use of food and nutritional supplements will aid the prevention of morbidity and mortality associated with several key contemporary illnesses. Nutrition knowledge changes with new scientific evidence, and health professionals must be aware of reliable sources of continuing education and information appropriate for themselves and their patients. Health care professionals have the responsibility to help our patients to synthesise new information without overlooking the most important thing: the need to follow a well-balanced diet.

2.8 References

1. Halsted CH. The relevance of clinical nutrition education and role models to the practice of medicine. *Eur J Clin Nutr* 1999; 53(Suppl 2): S29–34
2. Lawson M, Thomas M. Low vitamin D status of Asian 2 year olds living in England. *BMJ* 1999; 318: 28
3. Mera SL. Diet and disease. *Br J Biomed Sci* 1994; 51: 189–206
4. Willett WC. Diet and health: what should we eat? *Science* 1994; 264: 532–537
5. Doll R, Peto R. The causes of cancer quantitative estimates of avoidable risks of cancer in the United States today. *J Natl Cancer Inst* 1981; 66: 1191–1308
6. Willett WC. Diet, nutrition and avoidable cancer. *Environ Health Perspect* 1995; 103(Suppl 8): 165–170
7. Ferguson LR. Prospects for cancer prevention. *Mutat Res* 1999; 428: 329–338
8. Maxwell SR, Lip GY. Free radicals and antioxidants in cardiovascular disease. *Br J Clin Pharmacol* 1997; 44: 307–317
9. Berenson GS, Srinivasan SR, Nicklas TA. Atherosclerosis: a nutritional disease of childhood. *Am J Cardiol* 1998; 82(Suppl 10B): 22T-29T
10. Connor SL, Connor WE. Are fish oils beneficial in the prevention and treatment of coronary artery disease. *Am J Clin Nutr* 1997; 66(Suppl 4): 1020S–1031S
11. Department of Health. Nutrition and bone health: With particular reference to vitamin D and calcium. Report on health and social subjects 49. London: The Stationery Office, 1998
12. Fortin PR, Lew RA, Liang MH et al. Validation of a meta-analysis: the effects of fish oil in rheumatoid arthritis. *J Clin Epidemiol* 1995; 48: 1379–1390
13. Clarke R, Daly L, Robinson K et al. Hyperhomocysteinaemia: an independent risk factor for vascular disease. *N Engl J Med* 1991; 324: 1149–1155
14. Brattstrom LE. Vitamins as homocysteine lowering agents. *J Nutr* 1996; 126: 1276S–1280S
15. Graham IM, Daly LE, Refsum HM et al. Plasma homocysteine as a risk factor for vascular disease. The European Concerted Action Project. *JAMA* 1997; 277: 1775–1781
16. Gray DP. Dietary advice in British General Practice *Eur J Clin Nutr* 1999; 53(Suppl 2): S3–8
17. Buttriss JL. Food and nutrition: attitudes, beliefs, and knowledge in the United Kingdom. *Am J Clin Nutr* 1997; 65: 1985S–1995S
18. Goldberg JP. Nutrition and health communication: the message and the media over half a century. *Nutr Rev* 1992; 50: 71–77
19. Davison K. The quality of dietary information on the World Wide Web. *Clin Perform Qual Health Care* 1997; 5: 64–66
20. Moore H, Adamson AJ, Gill T, Waine C. Nutrition and the Health Care Agenda: A Primary Care perspective. *Fam Pract* 2000; 17: 197–202
21. Guidelines for dentists from the Department of Health. National Diet and Nutrition Survey. Report of the oral health survey. HMSO, 1998
22. Ashley JM, Jarvis WT. Position of the American Dietetic Association: food and nutrition misinformation. *J Am Diet Assoc* 1995; 95: 705–707
23. Schwartz NE, Borra ST. What do consumers really think about dietary fat? *J Am Diet Assoc* 1997; 97(Suppl 7): S73–75

24. Morris SE, Lean ME, Hankey CR, Hunter C. Who gets what treatment for obesity? A survey of GPs in Scotland. *Eur J Clin Nutr* 1999; 53 (Suppl 2): S44–48
25. Singer AJ, Werther K, Nestle M. Improvements are needed in hospital diets to meet dietary guidelines for health promotion and disease prevention. *J Am Diet Assoc* 1998; 98: 639–641
26. Davison C. Nutrition in nurse education (abstract). *Proceedings of the Nutrition Society* 1999; 58: 146A
27. Scott L, Belton EA. Attitudes of nutrition nurses to their role, to nutrition education and to relationships with dieticians (abstract). *Proceedings of the Nutrition Society* 1999; 58: 145A
28. Kushner RF. Barriers to providing nutrition counseling by physicians: a survey of primary care practitioners. *Prev Med* 1995; 24: 546–552
29. Helman A. Nutrition and general practice: an Australian perspective. *Am J Clin Nutr* 1997; 65 (Suppl 6): 1939S–1942S
30. Cadman L, Findlay A. Assessing practice nurses' change in nutrition knowledge following training from a primary care dietitian. *J R Soc Health* 1998; 118: 206–209
31. Campbell MK, DeVellis BM, Strecher VJ et al. Improving dietary behavior: the effectiveness of tailored messages in primary care settings. *Am J Public Health* 1994; 84: 783–787
32. Hariri S, Goodyer L, Anderson C, Meyer J. Cardio*Pharm*: interactive multimedia health promotion software for community pharmacy. *Nutrition and Food Science* 1997; 2: 71–75
33. McKie L, Clark GM, MacLellan M, Skerratt S. The promotion of healthy eating: food availability and choice in Scottish island communities. *Health Educ Res* 1998; 13: 371–382
34. Chandra RK. Effect of vitamin and trace-element supplementation on immune responses and infection in elderly subjects. *Lancet* 1992; 340: 1124–1127
35. McLauchlan WR, Sanderson J, Williamson G. Antioxidants and the prevention of cataracts. *Biochem Soc Trans* 1995; 23: 257S
36. Ellis JM, McKully KS. Prevention of myocardial infarction by vitamin B6. *Res Commun Mol Pathol Pharmacol* 1995; 89: 208–220
37. Teresi ME, Morgan DE. Attitudes of healthcare professionals toward patient counseling on drug-nutrient interactions. *Ann Pharmacother* 1994; 28: 576–580
38. Lasswell AB, DeForge BR, Sobal J, Muncie HL Jr, Michocki R. Family medicine residents' knowledge and attitudes about drug-nutrient interactions. *J Am Coll Nutr* 1995; 14: 137–143
39. Royal College of Physicians. Osteoporosis: clinical guidelines for strategies to prevent and treatment. London: Royal College of Physicians, 1999
40. Center JR, Nguyen TV, Schneider D, Sambrook PN, Eisman JA. Mortality after all major types of osteoporotic fracture in men and women: an observational study. *Lancet* 1999; 353: 878–882
41. Cooper C, Campion G, Melton LJ. Hip fractures in the elderly: a world-wide projection. *Osteoporosis International* 1992; 2: 285–289
42. Weaver CM. Calcium bioavailability and its relation to osteoporosis. *Proceedings of the Society for Experimental Biology and Medicine* 1992; 200: 157–160
43. MAFF, Ministry of Agriculture, Fisheries and Food. The dietary and nutritional survey of British adults – Further Analysis. London: HMSO, 1994
44. Lloyd T, Andon MB, Rollings N, Martel JK, Landis JR, Demers LM, Kieselhorst K, Kulin HE. Calcium supplementation and bone mineral density in adolescent girls. *JAMA* 1993; 270: 841–844
45. Chan GM, Hoffman K, McMury M. Effects of dairy products on bone and body composition in pubertal girls. *J Pediatrics* 1995; 126: 551–556
46. Cadogan J, Eastell R, Jones N, Barker ME. Milk intake and bone mineral acquisition in adolescent girls: randomised, controlled intervention trial. *BMJ* 1997; 315: 1255–1260
47. Nowson CA, Green RM, Hopper JL et al. A co-twin study of the effect of calcium supplementation on bone density during adolescence. *Osteoporosis International* 1997; 7: 219–225
48. Nordin BEC. Calcium and osteoporosis. *Nutrition* 1997; 13: 664–689
49. Nieves JW, Komar L, Cosman F, Lindsay R. Calcium potentiates the effect of estrogen and calcitonin on bone mass: review and analysis. *Am J Clin Nutr* 1998; 67: 18–24
50. Sikora K. Developing a global strategy for cancer. *Eur J Cancer* 1999; 35: 24–31

3 Nutrient Requirements in Health and Disease

Judith K. Donnelly

3.1 Introduction

In addressing his 'medical brethren' in the preface to the 1858 publication *Nutrition in Health and Disease,* eminent physician James Henry Bennet, wrote:

'My object in writing the following work has been to draw attention, forcibly, to the fact, constantly overlooked, that the imperfect performance of the digestive and nutritive functions leads, slowly but surely, to ill-health, to disease and to death.' [1].

Today, the study of eating and the absorption and assimilation of nutrients from food continues to engage the minds of research scientists and health professionals. A great deal of knowledge has been accumulated and applied with good effect since Bennet observed the need to study '*dietetics in connection with physiology and chemistry*'. This chapter considers how our knowledge of nutrition has been used to prevent disease, maintain health and promote well-being throughout life.

3.2 What Nutrients are Needed, and How Much?

Healthy nutrition requires the appropriate intake of energy from macronutrients (chiefly carbohydrate and fat) and adequate intake of essential amino acids (in the form of protein), essential fatty acids, vitamins and minerals. To support normal growth and metabolism the human body must obtain regular supplies of each nutrient from the diet or from body stores. If the supply of a particular nutrient becomes depleted, either through diet or illness, a deficiency state will develop. Conversely, an excess of particular nutrients may also be associated with ill-health.

In the past, in order to avoid nutrient deficiencies among the population, the UK government developed recommended daily intakes (RDIs, set in 1969) and then recommended daily amounts (RDAs, set in 1979) for each nutrient. However in dietary analysis RDA values can be easily misinterpreted, because the values are set high enough to meet the needs of almost every healthy person in the country. Thus the average person, and indeed the vast majority in the population, would be healthy consuming much less than the RDA value. High intakes of some nutrients may have undesirable effects.

Nutritional scientists, including epidemiologists, now seek to assess not only what levels of individual nutrients are required to prevent deficiency and maintain health in the population, but what levels might be regarded as appropriate for *optimal* health at various stages in the life cycle. This more sophisticated concept of optimum nutrition is a relatively recent development, and through its use scientists hope to reduce the risk of development of chronic diseases and optimise physiological and mental function, through dietary modification. Towards this end, in 1991 in the UK dietary reference values (DRVs) were published [2] providing information about requirements of individual nutrients; they were proposed on the basis of the evidence available, and they are in use today, guiding dietitians and other health professionals on the quality of diets.

3.3 Dietary Reference Values

The physiological requirement for each nutrient will depend to some extent on the individual's genetic and metabolic characteristics and may alter, for example due to changes in levels of activity or changes in overall composition of the diet. It is usually not practical for health professionals to determine the nutrient requirements of individuals and therefore the average requirements of similar groups of people are estimated. This approach has been used by the Panel on Dietary Reference Values of the Committee on Medical Aspects of Food Policy at the Department of Health to produce the information currently used by nutritionists and dieticians in the UK [2]. The DRV tables (see [3]) list the requirements for energy and for 33 individual nutrients, for the UK population, grouped by age and gender (and by stage of pregnancy or lactation status for women). The DRV figures are given as estimated *average* requirements (EAR), with additional figures for the majority of nutrients (representing +/– 2 standard deviations) indicating the reference nutrient intake level (RNI) and the lower reference nutrient intake level (LRNI). These latter levels are the requirement figures to meet the needs of 97.5% and 2.5% of the population respectively. Thus EAR, RNI and LRNI figures are used for guidance on the adequacy of the diets for groups of the population, rather than the whole population. When the figures are used to assess the diet of an individual, care must be taken in the comparisons because the intake levels of an individual are unlikely to match exactly with the needs determined for a particular group due to the variation in individual physiological requirements.

3.4 Meeting the Targets

In the UK today most people have reasonable access to good quality food and the symptoms of the classic deficiency diseases, such as beriberi and scurvy, are rarely seen. In general, whilst people do not have sufficient knowledge to assess their nutritional requirements, most seem to manage to obtain a diet sufficiently varied to prevent signs of severe deficiencies. However, there is much evidence of ill-health from poorly balanced diets, linked to the over-consumption of sugar, salt and fatty foods, often at the expense of fruit and vegetables. To encourage consumption of a varied diet, models are used for the purpose of illustration. One example is the plate model, developed by the Health Education Authority in 1994 [4]. This model features the visual image of a dinner plate with 5 approximate fractions occupied by examples from each of five food groups (fruit and vegetables about 33%, bread, cereals and potatoes also 33%, meat, fish and alternatives, such as pulses, 12%, milk and dairy foods 15%, fatty and sugary foods 8%).

Despite such health education developments, adverse socio-economic factors have a substantial influence on diet and there is a greater prevalence of diet-related ill-health in social classes IV and V. In some of the low-income subgroups of the population, the effects of under-nutrition may still impair growth and development in children and result in poor health and greater susceptibility to infection because of a lower immune function. Particularly vulnerable groups in the population are young children, adolescents, pregnant women and older adults. The 1998 report of the *Independent Inquiry on Inequalities in Health* chaired by Sir Donald Acheson [5] urged that a high priority be given to the health of women of childbearing age, expectant mothers and young children. Improving the diet of girls and women is likely to improve not only their own health, but more significantly that of their children throughout their lives, as discussed later in this chapter.

Inappropriate food choices amongst the more affluent majority in the population may also result in increased risk of chronic disease. Concerns include whether the diet meets the physiological requirements the various stages through life. If the diet at a particular stage in life is inadequate, even in respect of only one nutrient, this may lead to consequences later in life. For example, poor calcium intake through their adolescent and early adult years (and hence lower peak bone mass, achieved in early adulthood) may result in osteoporosis in older women. Osteoporosis occurs as a result of an age-related reduction in bone density, especially after the menopause, when the rate of loss is accelerated.

Even among the better educated and the more health conscious sectors of UK society, failure, or fear of failure to meet nutrition requirements because of lifestyle demands is commonly encountered. Such concern may arise from publicity of the national statistics indicating the prevalence of diet-related diseases. For example, a report on the prevalence of cardiovascular disease and its risk factors, based on the 1998 annual health survey and comparisons with the corresponding 1994 statistics, indicates that the prevalence of both coronary heart disease and stroke increased over this four year period [6]. Whilst increased life expectancy and birth control have resulted in a rise in the proportion of elderly in the population, the so-called 'diseases of affluence' including cardiovascular diseases, diet-related cancers, diabetes and hypertension are leading causes of morbidity and mortality and continue to drain health resources. Obesity may increase the chance of developing coronary heart disease (CHD), stroke and other chronic diseases including diabetes, hypertension and arthritis. The proportion of adult men and women who are obese (BMI >30) had doubled over the past twenty years to approximately 17% of men and 21% of women [6]. Hypertension is also a major predictor of CHD and is the most important risk factor for stroke, which along with other circulatory diseases are responsible for 200,000 deaths per annum in the UK [7].

Government health targets for the UK include substantial reductions in the death rate in people less than 75 years old from heart disease, strokes and cancers by 2010 [7]. Achieving these health outcomes demands that nutritionists and dieticians impress upon those responsible for health policies and the public that good nutrition is important at every stage in life. The following sections consider the influence of diet on health at the various stages through the life span and selected examples illustrate how health problems, which may be chronic and possibly fatal, are associated with under-nutrition or inappropriate food choices at stages through life.

3.5 Pregnancy and Lactation – Life-Long Health Implications of Nutrition

The nutritional status of the mother before and during pregnancy influences her fertility, the development of the fetus and the development of the breast-fed infant. For example, in underweight women, there is a close relationship between maternal bodyweight and that of the infant [8]. This relationship is of concern, because neonatal birth weight is the strongest predictor of infant morbidity and mortality [9]. During the period of the pregnancy and early childhood, the rate of growth of the child is remarkable, and is accompanied by many physiological and developmental changes.

Pregnancy and the initial post-natal months are particularly critical times for the growth and development, and good nutrition is essential. The effects on growth, body composition and body function of nutritional factors during fetal and early development are not restricted to the short-term. Early diet has long-term effects on development of sensory and cognitive abilities as well as on behaviour, and on mortality risks during adulthood. This phenomenon is a function of so-called 'programming' whereby the nutritional, hormonal and metabolic environment afforded by the mother may permanently 'programme' the structure, physiology and metabolism of the offspring [10].

Undernutrition of the fetus, whether from inadequate food intake by the mother, or inadequate transport or transfer of nutrients, leads to changes in gene expression resulting in these permanent, deleterious changes. Early infant feeding is related to insulin-dependent diabetes [11] and to cognitive development [12, 13] in older children. The long-term effects of undernutrition during the critical period of early development are also evident in adulthood and even in the next generation.

Many researchers, including Professor David Barker of the MRC Environmental Epidemiology Unit, have noted a strong association between low birth weight and risks of development of CHD in later life [10]. The weight at one year of age is also strongly associated with subsequent death rates from CHD in men: in their study Barker and colleagues noted that death rates fall steeply from those who were small at one year of age to those who were large [14]. Ravelli et al. [15] have suggested that the prevalence of obesity in adulthood is related to fetal and infant nutrition. Barker [10] argues that the long-term effects of fetal and infant nutrition can also be seen in the risks of diabetes, hypertension and risk of hypercholesterolaemia in adults. Barker [16] reported that studies in the UK, on people living in Sheffield, in Preston and in Hertfordshire showed that adults who were small as babies have raised blood pressure, raised serum cholesterol and plasma fibrinogen concentrations and impaired glucose tolerance. These are all risk factors for CHD.

The long term influence of fetal nutrition on physiology and metabolism are well illustrated by observations following the 'Dutch Hunger Winter' towards the end of World War II [17]. During the harsh winter of 1944 food supplies to parts of Holland were scarce because of a blockade; this led to severe calorie restrictions for the citizens. The baby girls conceived in western Holland during the famine, but born after liberation, were of normal birth weight, although decades later their own babies were born with low birth weights. It was concluded that the ability of the women to deliver nutrients to their own offspring was impaired by the physiological and metabolic consequences her undernutrition in the uterus.

The examples mentioned above demonstrate very clearly that undernutrition of the fetus has life-long outcomes and influences the health of subsequent generations. This issue is addressed in the report *Independent Inquiry into Inequalities in Health* [5] which underlines the influence of poverty on diet and emphasises the importance of improving the health of women of childbearing age. Research by Doyle and her co-workers in Hackney, an inner-city London borough, demonstrated that with few exceptions, low birth weight babies are born to women with exceptionally poor diets [18]. In considering the influence of socio-economic class, the main differences in the dietary intake of the lower socio-economic class pregnant mothers in the Hackney study with those of higher classes was not in the energy content, but in the consumption of protein, vitamins and minerals. In particular consumption of B group vitamins correlated with social class and with birth weight outcome. In the Hackney study intake of folate, which is found in fruit and green vegetables, correlated more strongly with socio-economic class than any other nutrient.

Although the influence of the maternal diet in the fetal development in undernourished women is widely accepted, the debate about the influence of diet on fetal development in well-nourished pregnant women continues. Mathews and co-workers [19] recently investigated the influence of maternal nutrition on the outcome of pregnancy using a prospective cohort study. The study was conducted using women recruited from antenatal clinics at a hospital on the south coast of England. The research team studied the effects of the diet on birth weight and on placental weight at birth. They reported that placental weight and birth weight were not associated with intake of any of the macronutrients. Although some micronutrients (vitamin C, vitamin E and folate) were positively associated with birth weight, this occurred only before adjustments were made for maternal height and smoking in the multivariate analysis undertaken. It seems that the discussion on the influence of diet on fetal development in well-nourished pregnant women is set to continue.

Folic acid is one example of a micronutrient whose influence on fetal development is now well known and is explained in detail elsewhere in this book. Dietary supplementation with folates around the periconceptual period to reduce the occurrence of neural tube defects in the fetus is the subject of health promotion campaigns. The potential advantages of supplementing the diet with other micronutrients at the stage of early pregnancy are less well identified. Nevertheless, given the increased demand for nutrients, the potential for insufficient intake is high amongst pregnant women with poor diets. In their comprehensive review article, Koletzko et al. [9] argue that greater knowledge about optimal supply of nutrients and other 'functional' food ingredients during fetal development and early childhood could lower the risks of ill-health throughout life and improve the chances of children realising their genetic potential. In order to work toward optimising early nutrition, the roles of protein and the micronutrients must be considered.

During pregnancy, women build up a store of approximately 2–4 kilograms of fat in their bodies to support the energy requirements of lactation. In addition to use of energy contained within these fat stores, extra energy must be obtained daily from the postpartum diet to support breast-feeding. The proportion of ingested nutrients available for milk synthesis depends on the nutrient stores and therefore on the maternal dietary intake. There is an association between maternal dietary intake and infant milk intake. The composition of the milk, particularly with regard to the content of the essential fatty acids, varies according to the type and quality of the maternal diet. In addition to the increased energy demand to support breast-feeding, there is an increased protein requirement, which in well-nourished new mothers will be readily supplied from the general increase in the size of the normal dietary intake. The vitamin and mineral requirements will also be usually met by a general increase in dietary intake, although the calcium demand is exceptionally high. If dietary intake of calcium is not sufficient, then the lactating mother's bones may begin to be demineralised to meet the demand, leading to the possibility of osteoporosis in the mother in her later years.

In the first few days after birth the milk produced is colostrum, providing both nutrients and immunological factors including antibodies that are protective against infection in the first few months of life. This is one of the many reasons why breast-feeding is strongly encouraged over bottle-feeding with formula milk. Five types specific antibodies, or immunoglobulins, are produced, with the IgA class being predominant. The lactating mother secretes very high levels of IgA into the colostrum to prevent pathogens attaching to the mucosal surfaces of the infant's gut. A second reason is that human milk contains the essential fatty acids (*n*-3 and *n*-6) and their longer chain derivatives including docosahexanoic acid (DHA), whereas conventional formula milks contain the essential fatty acids but only trace amounts, if any DHA [20]. There is a great deal of debate on whether the nutritional needs of babies can be met by the precursor essential fatty acids, or whether the long chain polyunsaturated fatty acid derivatives found in breast milk, such as DHA are also required in the diet (because the conversion to the derivatives occurs too slowly for optimal growth and development). The omega-3 long chain polyunsaturated fatty acid DHA

(22: 6 n-3) is believed to help the functions of the brain and central nervous system of the infant to develop rapidly during the third trimester of pregnancy and the initial months after the birth. The fetal brain undergoes neuroblast development during the first trimester and nerve glial development occurs in the third trimester, continuing into the first year of life. Nutritional deficiency at this critical period leads to psychomotor retardation, with long-term consequences.

In addition to long chain polyunsaturated fatty acids, other components of breast milk, for example hormones and growth factors may be important in neurological development [21]. Several studies into intelligence of bottle vs. breast fed infants have indicated that, especially if born prematurely, breast fed children perform better in tests of development or cognition, verbal ability or school performance as infants [21–23] and at 8 years of age [24]. Using data from studies published over 30 years, a meta-analysis of differences in cognitive development between breast-fed and formula-fed children, conducted by Anderson and colleagues [25] found that breast-feeding was associated with significantly higher scores for cognitive development.

3.6 The Weaning Process

The majority of lactating mothers can produce enough milk to meets the needs of their infant at the four months stage. By the time that the birth weight has doubled, at about six months of age, the quantity of breast milk that can be produced no longer supplies sufficient energy, protein, iron, zinc and vitamins A and D. Therefore weaning must occur for further development of the child. It is usual for babies to receive a milk-only diet up to 3 months old, then to receive additional semi-solid food and gradually more solid food at 6–9 months in a mixed diet until fully weaned. The main recommendation of The Department of Health's guidelines on weaning [26] is that solid foods should not be introduced until the baby is 4–6 months old, whether the baby is breast or bottle-fed. There is much concern that this guideline is not followed by the majority of mothers [27]. Early weaning may be associated with obesity, infection, adverse reactions to food, respiratory illness and cardiovascular disease [28]. This association is illustrated in a follow-up study of a cohort of 500 seven year-olds in Dundee by Wilson and colleagues [29]. In the study it was found that the children who had been weaned before 15 weeks of age were significantly heavier and fatter than those (of the same sex) who were introduced to solids later. The authors also noted that exclusive breast feeding for at least 15 weeks was associated with a significant reduction in respiratory illness during the first seven years of life and that early weaning was associated with the development of childhood wheezing.

The Department of Health's guidelines on weaning also recommend that a mixed diet should be offered to babies by 6 months of age. Late weaning may be associated with poor growth, a delay in pyschomotor and emotional development and iron-deficiency anaemia (see [26]). By 6 months of age the baby's sources of iron, accumulated in the uterus, have depleted and breast milk is a poor source of iron. It is important that the weaning diet contains good sources of iron, which may be obtained from foods such as red meat. In the UK iron deficiency anaemia is the most commonly reported nutritional disorder in early childhood, especially in poorly nourished young children and such a deficiency may be associated with psychomotor impairment. During the weaning process the other nutrients which are mostly likely to be inadequate in a poor diet are the essential fatty acids, essential amino acids, calcium, zinc and vitamins A and D [28]. In addition to being rich in these micronutrients, weaning foods should be rich in energy. The diet should not be modified to lower the fat content by inclusion of low fat foods before 2 years of age.

Babies should be receiving a wide variety of foods, distinguished by taste and texture, before they are one year old. Studies on home-prepared weaning foods have found that they may be too low both in energy and nutrients already mentioned; they often have high amounts of fibre (or non-starch polysaccharides, NSP), starch and protein [30]. In the diet of young children fruit and vegetable consumption should be encouraged. However, the diet should not be entirely based on plant foods rich in NSP [26]; there are several disadvantages including the possibility of diarrhoea, and the increased bulk causing a lowering of the energy density of the diet and so reducing the bioavailability of iron and zinc. From their survey of mothers regarding good infant feeding practices, Morgan and colleagues [31] noted that 95% of the mothers were aware of the importance of feeding a wide variety of foods and 76% did rate 'plenty of calories' as important. However, more than 80% of the mothers falsely believed that the infant's diet should be high in fibre (83%) and low in fat (88%). Reviewing the survey [28], Morgan comments 'These attitudes towards infant feeding habits were fortunately not achieved in the preparation of the diet'. Nevertheless this survey and others indicate that there is a clear need to educate mothers on good infant feeding practice: for example, on the fact that when using cows milk, whole milk rather than skimmed or semi-skimmed is the most appropriate choice of drink for children under 2 years.

3.7 Childhood

During childhood the pattern of growth and development continues to be influenced by a number of factors including heredity, hormones and the environment; and as appropriate nutrition is critical in this period, correct dietary intake is essential. As for babies, relative to their body weight, the pre-school and school child's requirement for energy, protein and micronutrients is greater than that of adults, because of the need to support rapid growth and development in addition to the requirements for basal metabolism and physical activity. From infancy through to puberty, the energy and nutrient requirements per kilogram bodyweight decline as the rate of growth decelerates with age.

With regard to fat and carbohydrate content of the diet, human breast milk provides a baby with 54% of its energy in the form of fat, contains simple sugars rather than starch, and does not contain NSP. The dietary recommendations for adults and older children are to consume less than 35% of calories in the form of fat, and less than 11% as non-milk extrinsic sugars, to eat 18 g per day of NSP and obtain more energy from starch, at the expense of sugars and fat. During the pre-school years the diet must be gradually modified from that required for infant growth, development and health to that which is more appropriate for adulthood.

To provide the child with the nutrients that will ensure proper growth and development, and benefit their future health, the diet must be balanced. This is achieved with foods containing protein and starchy foods (including wholegrain cereals) and fruit and vegetables and foods that are rich in micronutrients such as iron, zinc, calcium and vitamins A, C and D. However, the young child's diet should not contain too much NSP, to avoid the difficulties associated with obtaining sufficient energy and nutrients from a bulky, low energy-dense diet. It is important to encourage children to eat a variety of foods to avoid the possibility of nutritional deficiency. The Department of Health [26] recommend that the diet is supplemented with vitamin drops (A, C and D) where appropriate to avoid deficiency in the transition period from weaning to eating a diet that meets the adult guidelines at the age of 5 years.

In a national study, the National Diet and Nutrition Survey of $1^1/_2$–$4^1/_2$ year-olds [32] it was found that pre-school children in Britain were eating insufficient fruit and vegetables and iron-rich foods; 1 in every 12 children was anaemic. Also, the children were eating large quantities of salt and sugar. There is sufficient salt in milk and weaning foods for infant requirements and given the suspicions that salt may contributes to hypertension in adults, it is believed that opportunities to develop a preference for salty foods should be limited.

As young children cannot eat large amounts at one sitting, snacks are needed in addition to three meals each day. Although it is important that sufficient calories are provided for growth and energy requirements, snack food items should be carefully chosen because excessive consumption of sugary foods may result in dental caries (decay) as well as obesity. In the National Diet and Nutrition Survey of the under-fives, 17% had dental caries. The published data from the survey indicates that children with dental caries had higher intakes of sugar confectionery and soft drinks. Since milk is cariostatic and provides many micronutrients including calcium, it is an important drink for young children. The Department of Health [26] recommends that pre-school children receive a minimum of $^1/_3$ litre of milk every day.

The over-consumption of foods which are high in fat, sugar or salt by children is discouraged by health professionals because an acquired preference for these food types may last throughout life and be associated with health problems in later years. Obese children are more likely to become obese adults, with associated risks of health problems such as cardiovascular disease. Recent studies on the prevalence of childhood obesity indicate that approximately 19% of five year olds are overweight and 7% are obese [33].

3.8 Younger Schoolchildren

To meet the nutrient demands of childhood, the Department of Health [26] recommends that the general adult guidelines for the total fat content of the diet (35% or less of food energy), <11% non-milk extrinsic sugars and plenty of starch and NSPs are followed by the age of five. DRV levels have been established for children according to age (and gender for energy) for individual nutrients.

The growth rate of pre-adolescent children is relatively slow, although growth occurs in spurts with a corresponding effect on the child's appetite. During the pre-adolescent phase children grow 10 cm. taller and gain 2.5 kg in weight per year. In this period calcium is deposited to support bone growth and fat deposits may be increased to provide energy for the pre-pubertal growth spurt, when there is a change in height, body shape and composition.

As children begin school at the age of five, their diet and eating patterns are increasingly influenced by factors apart from the family, including their peers and advertising. The general guidelines in The Department of Health's report on the Diets of British Schoolchildren [34] outlined the concerns regarding the diet of this age-group in the UK population. Children in low-income families are those most likely to have inadequate intakes of nutrients. Children show the same socio-economic class differences as their parents with regard to their diet and undernutrition of children from poor families is a major concern highlighted in the Acheson report on Inequalities in Health [5]. Children in these families consume the most chips, white bread, sugar and sweets with the least milk and fruit and vegetables.

3.9 Adolescence

During adolescence there is a rapid and substantial growth spurt toward adult composition and body-size. Boys enter puberty with one sixth of their body-weight as fat, but because of the deposition of lean muscle, the proportion of fat in the body decreases to one tenth. In contrast girls also begin puberty with one sixth of their body weight as fat, but this increases to one fourth by the end of the pubescent phase. Between the ages of 12 and 17 years boys grow an average of 26 cm. taller and gain 26 kg in weight. Girls gain averages of 23 cm in height and 21 kg in weight between the ages of 10 and 14 years [34a].

This extraordinary period of growth and development has a profound effect on nutritional requirements and hence on appetite. It is not surprising to realise that there is a relatively high demand for energy and nutrients in this period: during their adolescent period boys accumulate 200 mg/day of calcium in their skeletons, 0.5 mg/day iron and 2 g/day protein [34a]. The DRVs set by the Department of Health [2] take account of these needs, and for this reason the DRV levels for intake of energy (EAR) and calcium for 15–18 year olds exceed those for adults. The protein and iron requirement for teenage boys is also higher than for grown men. The dietary guidelines for the adolescent period should be met in the same manner as for the population as a whole, with a balance between the five main food groups as shown in the 'healthy plate' model discussed earlier.

In considering the diet of teenage girls and all women of child-bearing age, the menstrual loss of iron must be taken into account, so DRV levels have been set correspondingly higher than for males [2, 3]. The RNI value for iron intake of 14.8 mg/day for women is, by definition, sufficient to meet the needs of the majority of teenage girls and women, though for women with exceptionally heavy menstruation iron supplements may be appropriate. Teenage girls and women who are underweight and practice weight control through dietary restriction may experience a delay in the onset of menstruation and difficulties with sustaining menstruation cycles related to low amounts of body fat. If adolescent girls attempt to reduce their weight by dieting then insufficient intakes of many nutrients including iron, calcium may occur. In a study of schoolchildren in the East End of London, it was reported that one quarter of young teenage girls had levels of calcium, magnesium, iron, zinc and vitamin A and riboflavin below the LRNI levels [35].

Low calcium intakes in teenage girls are of particular concern because of the associated risk of osteoporosis in later life. Even a small increase in bone density results in a substantial reduction in the risk of fracture and so it is important to maximise bone density. During adolescence the rate of calcium accretion is highest, and calcium may be a limiting nutrient for optimum bone growth in teenage diets [35 a]. Dairy foods provide about 60% of the calcium in the UK diet and populations at risk of developing osteoporosis are those who do not consume sufficient dairy products. Osteoporosis affects not only older women who are oestrogen deficient after the menopause, but younger women, e.g. dancers and athletes with low oestrogen levels because they are underweight or training too much.

3.10 Adulthood

Healthy adulthood is dependent on nutrition in childhood. During adulthood there is no further growth, except for a small increase in bone mass (until the peak is reached in early adulthood), and increases in fat deposition. In the period of middleage, excess fat in an energy-dense diet and alcohol and an inactive lifestyle contribute to health problems.

The prevalence of hypertension has a positive correlation with obesity, sodium (salt) intake and alcohol consumption. Hypertension is also a major predictor of CHD and is the most important risk factor for stroke.

It is not only the percentage body fat that is important to health in adulthood, but also the distribution. In men and in post-menopausal women intra-abdominal (central) adiposity is considered to be a risk factor for cardiovascular disease and for non-insulin-dependent diabetes mellitus (NIDDM), a disease characterised by an increase in insulin resistance and poorer glucose tolerance. Although adult obesity may be associated with obesity in childhood, only one third of obese adults were overweight as children.

Adults are recommended to follow the DRV guidelines, paying attention to the contribution of fat (<35% of calories) and saturated fatty acids (<11% of energy intake) and polyunsaturated fatty acids (PUFA) composition of the dietary fat. At the population level, the current UK intake of fat is too high, at 39% of food energy [36], and it is not unusual for British adults to consume a diet in which >50% of the calories come from fat often containing a high proportion of saturated fatty acids.

The habitual consumption of diets rich in fats and saturated fatty acids predisposes the population to risks of CHD and certain types of cancer. There is epidemiological evidence for the 'lipid hypothesis' of CHD, which states that dietary fat consumption alters blood lipid levels and that elevated blood lipids exacerbate atherogenesis. The clinical symptoms of atheroscelosis include myocardial infarction and stroke. Certain dietary saturated fatty acids, including myristic acid, have a marked plasma cholesterol-raising effect and dietary cholesterol has a more modest effect. PUFA, including linoleic acid and monounsaturated fatty acids (MUFA, chiefly oleic acid) in the diet have a modest plasma cholesterol-reducing effect, though less potent than the elevating effect of some of the saturated fats. In adults with abnormally high plasma cholesterol levels (≥ 6 mM), cutting the total amount saturated fat and cholesterol-rich foods in the diet may reduce plasma cholesterol. However, the body can synthesise cholesterol and therefore restricting dietary cholesterol may only have a rather modest effect on blood lipid levels.

The major cholesterol carrying proteins are low-density lipoprotein (LDL) and high-density lipoprotein (HDL). The plasma LDL cholesterol concentration is a predictor of the risk of CHD, whereas HDL cholesterol concentration is inversely related to the risk. Recent evidence has suggested that there are specific and unique effects of individual fatty acids on plasma cholesterol and its distribution between the various lipoprotein classes. In the near future it seems likely that this knowledge will be used to consider the fatty acid profile of fats and oils to provide specific LDL cholesterol lowering dietary recommendations [37], though none are available at present.

3.11 Older Years

Nutritional requirements in later life are similar to those for younger adults and although energy needs are reduced because of a reduction in basal metabolic rate and in physical activity, there is no reduction in the requirements for most essential nutrients. The report on the Nutrition of Elderly People [38] recommended that the majority of people over 65 years maintain a diet similar to that for younger adults. The UK DRVs for nutrients for those over 50 years are given in the Department of Health's guide [2, 3].

Elderly people are at risk of poor nutrition as a consequence of the ageing process, an increased incidence of disease, and psychological and social factors, including poverty. (It is interesting to note that life expectancy at 65 years is 2.5 years greater for men in social classes I and II compared to social classes IV and V [5].)

Ageing is characterised by a decline in physiological function and changes in adult body composition. Changes in body composition which occur in old age in the 'healthy elderly' start with the menopause in women and continue until about 70 years of age. For men, similar, though less severe changes appear at about 60–70 years [39]. Total body water decreases from middle-age in men and from about 60 years in women. By 70 years of age, 40% of skeletal muscle mass has been lost compared with that in young adult life. However there may be an increase in body fat up until the age of 70–80 years, and therefore change in body weight and/or a change in shape, with increasing intra-abdominal deposition of body fat. As for other age groups obesity is a common problem and because of the excess weight, obese elderly people are likely to suffer from age-related conditions more severely, for example, cardio-respiratory problems and osteoarthritis of the knees.

Decreasing bone-mass in both men and women is one well known characteristic of old age. The process begins in middle age. Bone mineral and matrix disappear more rapidly than deposition of bone tissue and the rate of loss for women accelerates dramatically in the early post-menopausal years, about 5 years after the menopause. During this period bone mass may decrease at a rate of 3–5% per year [40] and osteoporosis, a condition of the reduced bone density, is the major underlying cause of fractures in the elderly. Older women in particular should avoid low calcium intakes by consuming dairy products to reduce the risk of osteoporosis and fracture. As vitamin D is essential for calcium absorption and utilisation, adequate dietary intake of this vitamin is necessary for the housebound elderly whose synthesis of vitamin in the skin is poor.

Immunocompetence also declines progressively with age, but varies between individuals and depends also on the quality of the diet. Lowered immunity is associated with a poor nutritional status and is linked to protein, zinc and vitamin levels. Protein-energy malnutrition results in impairment of cell-mediated immunity and the affinity of antibodies for antigens may be reduced. Alterations in protein metabolism and hence concentrations of the amino acid glutamine, produced by the immune system at times of stress, also lower the immune function: response to an infection may be impaired when glutamine levels are too low.

Cancer is associated with depressed immunocompetence and the decline in immune function with advancing age is linked to the development of cancer. Antioxidant nutrients, including β-carotene, vitamin C and vitamin E are believed to influence immunocompetence and cancer development. Interactions between nutritional status, the immune response and cancer are complex, but it is thought that antioxidant status may modulate the immune response in cancer. The over 85 s are the most vulnerable age group and also the group most likely to experience problems with diet.

Life expectancy depends on genetic, environmental and dietary factors. Death is inevitable and whilst the maximum human life span is around 120 years of age, few achieve this. However, many do live to 85 or more years of age. Older people in western countries (including the UK) often die of myocardial infarction or cancer. It may take many years for the accumulation of all the different changes in DNA within the body's cells that eventually result in the development of cancer, and with a few notable exceptions, for most cancers the rate of incidence rises very sharply with age. 30% of people have cancer by the age of 85 years of age [41].

3.12 Conclusion

In the 19th century, at the time when Bennet wrote the first edition of his book '*Nutrients in Health and Disease*', about a quarter of the children born died before the age of five and infectious diseases were the major cause of death in Britain, with one in every three deaths attributed to infection in the 1850s. Thanks to major advances in public health, including nutrition, infectious disease has become an insignificant cause of death in the UK.

In Britain today circulatory diseases are the most important cause of mortality. In England and Wales in 1999 the main causes of death were heart disease (21%) and cerebrovascular diseases (10%) with a further 25% of all deaths from all cancers [42]. Almost 90,000 people die each year before 65 years of age and of these 32,000 die of cancer and 25,000 of heart disease, stroke and related illnesses [43]. The fact that many of these deaths could be prevented is highlighted in the UK Government's published targets to reduce deaths from these causes [7]. Although these diseases are multifactorial in their aetiology, many of the deaths are related to poor diet, and many of the diseases are indeed 'the diseases of affluence'. Despite major improvement in the safety and quality of food and in diet, the concerns about diet related diseases and mortality are stronger than ever.

Even with our vast knowledge of human nutrition, much remains to be learnt, especially regarding public health nutrition. Achieving dietary change in the population represents a major public health challenge [7]. In developing appropriate strategies we should consider that perhaps some of our problems stem from the fact that our diet is increasingly influenced by psychological and socio-cultural factors at the expense of our physiological needs as we progress through our life span from birth to death.

It is interesting to consider Bennet's 19th century observation on the distinction between animals and human beings with regard to diet selection:

'Food contains the required chemical elements of nutrition in variable proportions, and instinct guides man and all animated beings in the choice of the kind of food required by his and their organisations. This instinct, however, may be and often is, marred or perverted in man. The food instinct is not so strong with him as it is with the brute creation, the members of which generally limit themselves to the kind of food upon which nature has intended him to live and thrive. Perhaps it is so because he has reason to guide and direct him. It therefore behoves man to make use of his reason, to study himself, and thus direct his appetites and food-desires.'

On entering the 21st century we still have much to learn about ourselves and nutrition, in health and disease.

3.13 References

1. Bennet JH. *Nutrition in health and disease: a contribution to hygiene and to clinical medicine*, 2nd edn. London, J and A Churchill, 1876
2. Department of Health. *Dietary reference values for food energy and nutrients for the United Kingdom*. London: HMSO (Report on Health and Social Subjects No. 41), 1991
3. Salmon J. *Dietary reference values: a guide; prepared for the Department of Health*. London: HMSO, 1991
4. Gatenby SJ, Hunt P, Rayner M. The National Food Guide: development of the dietetic criteria and nutritional characteristics. *J Hum Nutr Dietet* 1995; 8: 323–334
5. Department of Health. *Independent inquiry into inequalities in health: report*. London: The Stationery Office, 1998
6. Erens B and Primatesta P (eds). *Health survey for England: cardiovascular disease '98*. Vol. 1: Findings. London: The Stationery Office, 1999
7. Department of Health. *Saving lives: our healthier nation*. London: The Stationery Office, 1999
8. Luke B and Petrie RH. Intrauterine growth: correlation of infant birth weight and maternal postpartum weight. *Am J Clin Nutr* 1980; 33: 2311–2317
9. Koletzko B, Aggett PJ, Bindels JG et al. Growth, development and differentiation: a functional food science approach. *Br J Nutr* 1998; 80: S5-S45
10. Barker DJP. *Mothers, babies and disease in later life*, 2nd edn. London: Churchill Livingstone, 1994
11. Virtanen SM, Rasanen L, Aro A et al. Infant feeding in Finnish children >7 years of age with newly diagnosed IDDM. *Diabetes Care* 1991; 14: 415–417
12. Lucas A, Morley R, Cole TJ, Lister G and Leeson-Payne C. Breast milk and subsequent intelligent quotient in children born pre-term. *Lancet* 1992; 339: 261–264
13. Lanting C I, Fidler V, Huisman M, Touwen BCL, and Boersma ER. Neurological differences between 9 year-old children fed breast-milk or formula-milk as babies. *Lancet* 1994; 344: 1319–1322
14. Osmond C, Barker DJP, Winter PD, Fall CHD and Simmonds SJ. Early growth and death from cardiovascular disease in women. *BMJ* 1993; 307: 1519–1524
15. Ravelli GP, Stein ZA and Susser MW. Obesity in young men after famine exposure in utero and early infancy. *N Engl J Med* 1976; 295: 349–353
16. Barker D. The fetal and infant origins of adult disease: an overview. In: *The Growing Cycle, Mother and Child*. Proceedings of a conference held on 24 November 1994. London: National Dairy Council, pp9–16, 1994
17. Lumey LH. Decreased birth weights in infants after maternal in utero exposure to the Dutch famine of 1944–1945. *Paediatr Perinat Epidemiol* 1992; 6: 240–253
18. Doyle W. Preparing for pregnancy: which groups are the most vulnerable? In: *The Growing Cycle, Mother and Child*. Proceedings of a conference held on 24 November 1994. London: National Dairy Council, pp 17–26, 1994
19. Mathews F, Yudkin P, Neil A. Influence of maternal nutrition on outcome of pregnancy: prospective cohort study. *BMJ* 1999; 319: 339–43
20. Jenson RG, Ferris AM, Lammi-Keefe CJ. Lipids in human milk and infant formulas. *Annu Rev Nutr* 1992; 12: 417–441
21. Morley R. Food for the infant's brain. *BNF Nutrition Bulletin* 1998; 23: 65–76
22. Florey C du V, Leech AM, Blackhall A. Infant feeding and mental and motor development at 18 months of age in first born singletons. *Int J Epidemiol* 1995; 24: S21–26
23. Morley R, Cole TJ, Powell R, Lucas A. Mother's choice to provide breast milk and developmental outcome. *Arch Dis Child* 1988; 63: 1382–1385
24. Lucas A, Morley, R Cole TJ, Lister G, Leeson-Payne C. Breast milk and subsequent intelligence quotient in children born preterm. *Lancet* 1992; 339: 261–264
25. Anderson, JW, Johnston BM, Remley DT. Breast-feeding and cognitive development: a meta-analysis. *Am J Clin Nutr* 1999; 70: 525–535

26. Department of Health. *Weaning and the weaning diet*. London: HMSO (Report on Health and Social Subjects No. 45), 1994
27. Foster K, Lader D, Cheeseborough S (eds). *Infant feeding 1995: A survey of infant feeding practices in the UK carried out by Social Survey Division of ONS on behalf of the Department of Health*. London: The Stationery Office, 1997
28. Morgan J. Weaning: when and what. *BNF Nutrition Bulletin* 1998; 23: Suppl. 1, 35–45
29. Wilson AC, Forsyth JS, Greene SA, Irvine L, Hau C, Howie PW. Relation of infant diet to childhood health: seven year follow-up of a cohort of children in Dundee infant feeding study. *BMJ* 1998; 316: 21–25
30. Stordy BJ, Redfern A, Morgan JB. Healthy eating for infants – mothers' actions. *Acta Paediatr* 1995; 84: 733–741
31. Morgan JB, Redfern AM, Stordy B J. Healthy eating for infants – mothers' attitudes. *Acta Paediatr* 1995; 84: 512–515
32. Gregory JR, Collins DL, Davies PSW, Hughes JM and Clarke PC. *National Diet and Nutrition Survey of Children Aged $1^1/_2$–$4\ ^1/_2$ years*. London: HMSO (Report on Health and Social Subjects No. 36), 1995
33. Reilly JJ, Dorosty AR, Emmett PM. Prevalence of overweight and obesity in British children: cohort study. *BMJ* 1999; 319: 1039
34. Department of Health. *The diets of british schoolchildren*. London: HMSO, 1989

34a. Webb GP. Nutrition a health promotion approach. London: Edward Arnold, 1995

35. Doyle W, Jenkins S, Crawford MA, and Puvandendran K. The nutritional status of schoolchildren in an inner city area. *Arch Dis Child* 1994; 70: 376–381

35a. Cadogan J, Enotell R, Jones N, Barker ME. Milk intake and bone mineral acquisition in adolescent girls; randomised, controlled intervention trial. *BMJ* 1997; 315: 125–126

36. MAFF. *The National Food Survey 1998*. London, The Stationery Office, 1999
37. Mangiapane EH and Salter, AM. *Diet, Lipoproteins and Coronary Heart Disease – a Biochemical Perspective*. Nottingham University Press, 1999
38. Department of Health. *The nutrition of elderly people*. London: HMSO (Report on Health and Social Subjects No. 43), 1992
39. Chumlea WC, Vellas B and Guo SS. Malnutrition or healthy senescence. *Proc Nutr Soc* 1998; 57: 593–598
40. Cooper C. Osteoporosis – an epidemiological perspective: a review. *J R Soc Med* 1989; 82: 753–757
41. Ames BN. Endogenous oxidative DNA damage, ageing and cancer. *Free Rad Res Comms* 1989; 7: 121–128
42. Office for National Statistics. *Deaths, 1999 registrations: death by age, sex and underlying cause*. Extracted from Health Statistics Quarterly – 06. http://www.statistics.gov.uk/Statbase.2000
43. Department of Health. *Our healthier nation*. London: The Stationery Office, 1998

4 Placebo and Panacea: The Healing Effect of Nutritional Supplements

Nicholas W. Read

No less than forty per cent of the British population take regular nutritional supplements. Most take cod liver oil capsules and multivitamin tablets, but evening primrose oil, minerals and herbal remedies are also very popular. Nutrition supplements now constitute a multimillion pound industry. At the last estimate, the figure for the total cost of nutrition supplements had risen to an astounding 360 million pounds a year [1] and the market is set to increase for at least another four years. Self medication with supplements has increased in parallel with the use of alternative or complementary therapy. One in five Britons now use complementary therapies, while in the United States, there are more visits to providers of alternative medicine than to primary care physicians [2]. Similar trends are occurring throughout the developed world. For example between 25 and 75% of people living in the UK, Holland, Germany, Finland and Australia undertake some form of alternative or complementary therapy to treat the chronic malaise that orthodox medicine does not help. Japan spends one and a half billion dollars per year on herbal (kampo) remedies.

There seems little biological justification for such widespread use of nutritional supplements among people living in developed countries. Only the very old and infirm or those suffering from severe gastrointestinal disease causing malabsorption suffer symptoms of vitamin and mineral deficiencies. Nutritionists may argue that many people need supplements because modern western diets consist of 'fast' or 'convenience' foods that are unbalanced and deficient in micronutrients. This argument is difficult to sustain. The large amounts of meat that are consumed by most Western populations contain many of the vitamins and minerals that we need in ample quantities. Fruit drinks often contain added vitamin C and breakfast cereals, bread, fat spreads and many other foods are fortified with vitamins and minerals. In fact, the diet of Britain and other developed countries is more likely than ever before to contain all the nutrients we need in sufficient proportions for optimal health [3–5]. How else would we explain the secular increases in average height, weight and reproductive life span? It is not so much that nutrition in the population of most western countries is deficient, it is more that it is excessive. Obesity and the diseases that are associated with it are arguably the biggest nutritional problem in our overdeveloped society.

So what is going on? Why have so many people turned to self medication and alternative therapies? Are we really a sick society? Or have we become a race of hypochondriacs, who spend our time worrying about the illnesses we might get if we don't take supplements? And are we so disillusioned with the ability of our health care systems to look after us that we have to seek alternatives? There is some truth in all of these postulates.

The 40% of the population that consume nutritional supplements are not the elderly, the underweight, those sick with other illnesses, or those consuming an inadequate diet. As Kirk and Cade reported in a recent paper, 'there is evidence that many of those who use supplements do not actually need them to meet a deficiency of nutrients' and in addition 'supplement users are already health conscious' and have 'a high consumption of fruits and vegetables' [6, 7]. They might be characterised as the worried well or perhaps more accurately, the worried and unwell. They include middle aged people concerned about getting old, mothers worried about the health of their children, high pressure executives exhausted by the demands of their work, young people eager to attract a mate, those who are stressed out and need something to help them cope, and people with so called 'functional' illnesses that are difficult to diagnose and impossible to cure and strongly associated with emotional upset. For them, nutritional supplements seem to act as charms, talismans or amulets that ward off evil influences; psychobiological regulators that rectify emotional and visceral activity by conveying a feeling a safety and confidence. This in essence is the placebo or healing effect.

The purpose of this chapter is not so much to examine the scientific claims of various supplements; that has been done in other chapters in this book. It is more to examine the effects of supplements in a generic sense by exploring how belief in their efficacy causes people to feel better. There is certainly some biological justification for giving iron and folic acid supplements to pregnant women and those about to become pregnant, and perhaps for enhancing the diet of teenage girls with calcium, but does Vitamin E really improve your sex life and are megadoses of Vitamin C really a good idea to ward off winter colds? These and the claims for many other nutritional supplements do not stand up to scientific scrutiny. So should most supplements be dismissed as useless? This would seem counterproductive when so many people feel so much better taking them. Such beneficial outcomes, however, may have little to do with their biological effects but are probably related more to what particular supplements represent for the people taking them. If a person expects a supplement to make him better and this belief is endorsed by health professionals and by the media, then there is every chance that he will feel better [8]. It seems likely therefore that most nutritional supplements act as what are popularly known as placebos. In other words, they work by faith, by suggestion, tapping into the people's beliefs, reinforcing their expectations, restoring their self confidence and putting them in control of their own health. There is nothing wrong, duplicitous or substandard in this. It is, after all, the central component of healing. All devices used to treat or prevent disease must exert some placebo effect; the fact that they may also have a direct action on biological processes just enhances the 'patients' healing sense of confidence in the treatment.

'I know that just seeking and receiving treatment made me feel better, less disabled, less distressed, more hopeful – and this in turn may have speeded my recovery' [9].

It is important that we do not dismiss or underestimate the notion of faith or belief in the prevention and treatment of disease. Instead, we should seek to understand it better and use that knowledge responsibly to improve the health of our fragile society.

This chapter is divided into four sections. The first section will explore why so many people in our society feel unwell. The second considers the nature of the placebo effect and how it may be enhanced. The third argues why nutritional supplements make excellent placebos. And the final section discusses the ethics of prescribing and marketing placebos in the guise of nutritional supplements.

4.1 Why Do So Many People Feel Unwell

Feeling unwell does not necessarily imply that a person has an infection, a cancer or any other obvious biological illness, it is about feeling insecure, exhausted, hopeless, helpless, depressed, fragmented, angry, panicky and out of control. The nearest we can get to a definition may be to say that feeling unwell is a prolonged state of negative emotional tension. This may be a reaction to a physical illness but in many cases it is not. Emotional tension is generated by events that overwhelm or undermine our ability to cope and by situations in which our sense of integrity and self confidence is threatened. This happens when we are ill but it also happens when we run short of money, when our children leave home, our parents get ill and die, the company we are working for runs short of orders, our partner spends more and more time away from home, our marriage fails [10]. Tension is created in the conflict between the clinging to the familiar and needing to risk change; between holding on and letting go.

The term 'emotion' implies that which causes movement. It is what makes us change, adapt and grow to accommodate an ever increasing range of experience. If we dare not respond to the emotional imperative for fear of risking loss and disintegration, then we are left with the tension of indecision and the frustration of feeling trapped or stuck. This chronic state of tension, which is mediated by the sympathetic and parasympathetic nervous systems, may be discharged not only through emotional expressions of panic, anger and depression but also by physiological changes resulting in symptoms of tiredness, headaches, insomnia, bowel upsets, and indigestion. These physical symptoms are 'self protective because they divert attention from the 'impossible' situation causing the emotional tension and focus effort on the quest for a cure for the physical illness.

People with chronic anxiety, panic, depression and 'functional' somatic symptoms show impaired regulation of the physiological responses to threat, which are indicated by exaggerated or suppressed activity in the autonomic nervous system and the hypothalamo-pituitary-adrenal (HPA) Axis that secretes the stress hormone, cortisol [11]. Prolonged emotional tension does not just cause 'functional' symptoms, it can result in actual pathological change. The links between psychological tension and so called 'organic' disease is well documented in hypertension, peptic ulcers, ulcerative colitis, thyrotoxicosis and coronary heart disease. Such illnesses come to provide an identity, a sense of meaning for the patients suffering; something palpable and tangible, a valid reason for feeling ill and for seeking help that avoids the need to acknowledge the real reason for the emotional tension.

Psychological and functional symptoms are becoming much more common than they used to be. In the UK, symptoms that have no obvious pathological basis account for at least 20% of family doctor consultations and 35% of specialist referrals [12]. Similar figures exist for other western countries. But this is just the tip of the iceberg. Statistics indicate that 30 to 40% of people, living in the developed countries of the world suffer from chronic tiredness, 40% from dyspepsia, 15% from backache, 20% from chronic bowel disturbances, 20% from recurrent abdominal pain, 50% are overweight and 35% of young women suffer from severe premenstrual symptoms. Anxiety and depression affect 20% of women and 13% of men [13]. Literally, millions of people are tortured by headaches, racked by back pains, tormented by abdominal gripes and embarrassed by diarrhea. Ringing in the ears, exhaustion, sleep deprivation, constipation, debilitating nausea, faintness and anorexia are also common. Nearly half the population is overwhelmed by the burden of obesity. Many are terrified by shortness of breath or chest pain, or too anxious, too depressed and too sick to cope. But why is this?

The simple answer is that the lives of so many people living in our post-modern Western culture seem to lack that sense of consistency and stability that contains and processes emotional tensions. We appear to be a fragile society, out of kilter with the environment we have created for ourselves. In the early part of this century, people would marry life for life, bring up their family in the same home, work in the same job, and live in the same town until they died. Nowadays the average person living in many 'western countries' would expect to change jobs three or four times, marry twice and move home five times. At no time in our history has human society gone through a greater period of change with such unprecedented acceleration [14]. People no sooner get used to the emotional tension induced by one set of changes than another hits them. And like London buses, changes tend to come in groups. For example, a change in job can mean moving house, separation from family members. There is no time to reflect and come to terms with what is happening. More than ever before, people have to live with an existence that is unstable and unpredictable. The threat of marital disruption, job loss, moving house are always there, providing a constant undercurrent of emotional tension. The dramatic increases in the prevalence of functional disease and depression during the last forty years and demand for self medication may well reflect the difficulties that people have experienced in coming to terms with the changes in their lives.

People vary considerably according to how they respond to the same life events. Some seem to have the self confidence and emotional containment to deal with whatever life throws at them while others seem to panic and despair at the slightest turn of fortune. There are few people who would not experience a sense of fragmentation during marital separation or divorce, a loss of self confidence during unemployment, a sense of personal desecration after a violent or sexual attack, a dreadful emptiness after the death of a child. Such awful events would make most people ill. But some people are so vulnerable and on-the-edge that they may become unwell as a result of everyday events such as being ignored by an acquaintance or having an argument with a colleague. Many are constantly tormented by the ever present worry of old age, loneliness and illness. Such sensitive souls need the support of friends and family, the security of their home and marriage, the importance of their role in the workplace and the sense of identity conveyed by their possessions, the holidays they take, the causes they espouse, their faith, the football learn they support to reinforce their fragile integrity. Loss of any of these factors can leave them exposed to feelings of chaos and fragmentation.

Our ability to regulate our emotional responses is developed early in life through interaction with our parents [15,16]. The infant is born helpless into the world, reacting to changes in his environment with obvious physiological distress. His interaction with the environment has to be mediated and regulated in the first instance by his 'mother'[1], who not only feeds him, protects him, and keeps him warm and clean, but also provides the security and containment, in which basic biological rhythms of sleep and feeding and more complex repertoires of behaviour are inculcated by the aid of subtle signals such as smiling, gentle touch, modulation of speech and eye contact [17]. As the infant grows, he develops the mental space and self confidence with which to regulate his own physiological and behavioural responses through the consistency of the relationship with his parents. Slowly he learns to create a safe place in his mind, comforting himself with a piece of cloth or a cuddly toy, which he imbues with special meaning [18], and reassuring himself with nursery stories, with their images of family unity and recovery from danger. The relationship with father creates another viewpoint to take on board, while the spreading network of family and friends and ever increasing encounters with a wider world provide a multitude of perspectives and experience allow the growing personality to achieve sufficient emotional maturity, individuality and independence to deal confidently with the vicissitudes of human society.

The acquisition this space in the mind to think, to disarm threat by seeing it in perspective with insight and understanding based on life's experience so that it can be dealt with calmly and efficiently, is the secret of growing up into an independent and functional adult. It starts in infancy through the combination of a consistent relationship with parents and the allocation of tolerable absences and proceeds through relationships with a wider world. Failure of the relationship with his mother and/or the absence of a father can leave the 'grown up' child without sufficiently mental resources to cope calmly with the changes and adversities that affect us all and too dependant on external factors; possessions, family, friends, home, institutions and beliefs to hold the personality together.

[1] In this context and in the rest of the article, the term mother does not necessarily imply any genetic connection but means one who performs the mothering role, is the primary cater in the person's early life. I realise this is not always the case. Some fathers have primary responsibility for their children from birth and there may be nannies, childminders and relatives who perform the mothering role. Similarly, the term father is used to denote the role of the father in providing another perspective and a conduit to an engagement with a wider world. Finally, I have also chosen for the sake of simplicity to use the word he as a general personal pronoun even though there is at least a 50% chance it could be 'she'.

The subsequent loss of any of these factors can leave the personality exposed to raw feelings and tensions, which may be expressed through anxiety, disturbed behaviour and visceral upset. In metaphorical terms, the hero is left at the mercy of his demons, which make him ill and can only be banished by the use of magic charms or spells. Immature thinking is notoriously black and white.

The demands of work, the erosion of family ties, the fragmentation of societal structures have made it increasingly difficult for modern parents to get it right. Fathers may not be around enough to form the vital other relationship with their developing infant and provide a containing environment for the family. Mothers feel unsupported and struggle to cope. Some may abandon their infants in front of the television and placate them with food and treats while they get on with the jobs that need to be done. Others may overcompensate, shielding their infant and themselves from the harsh realities of independence by doing everything for them. In either way, the child does not get the social environment he needs to develop the emotional maturity to become fully independent. As the psychoanalyst, Eric Brenman put it, a mother, who is unsupported and feels she may not cope, communicates that anxiety to her infant and provides a tense and erratic environment. At the same time, she tries to deny psychic reality and avoid the catastrophe she creates by placating her infant with treats and toys [19]. Such a child may become a fragile and vulnerable adult who can easily feel overwhelmed with modem life and needs help from medicines and nutritional supplements just to keep body and soul together.

This existential sense of fragility is exacerbated by the undermining of the institutions that made up structure of our society and provided a sense of safety and containment. The authority of The Church, 'The Government', 'The Monarchy', 'The Law', 'The National Health Service', and 'The Family' has undergone a steady erosion in the last fifty years. This has left a vacuum in which vulnerable and insecure people flounder around looking for some sense of meaning in their lives, a code of ethics, a model of behaviour, a basis for belief and attitude. Nature and society abhors a vacuum and so the space is being filled by the all powerful mass information media. But instead of providing a focus of stability, the television, radio, magazines and the Internet generate messages that are confusing, contradictory, sensationalist and at times quite irresponsible. Far from being contained, our insecurities are fuelled by the idea, promulgated by the media, that no aspect of our modern life is without threat. The food we eat, the water we drink, the air we breathe, the cars we drive, the work we do, the sex we enjoy, even the phones we use; all are potentially dangerous and can shorten our lives, sometimes quite dramatically, or so the media would have us believe. We are constantly alarmed by the risks to our health caused by aspects of living that we tend to take for granted. With the reputation of the medical profession at an all time low, no wonder so many people are turning to alternative or complementary therapies and to nutritional supplements to keep them going.

4.2 The Placebo or Healing Effect

If disease or fears of disease are caused by tensions related to difficulties in coping with life situations, then it stands to reason that anything that calms these tensions and restores a feeling of self confidence will make the person feel better. The 'Placebo Effect' underlines the importance of faith and confidence in healing. Placebos work by suggestion [20]. They are medicine at the level of the idea. The recipient has faith in the therapeutic idea, and the ensuing feelings of self confidence and control normalise the activities of the sympathetic and parasympathetic nervous systems and the HPA axis, reducing emotional tension and restoring visceral function [11, 21].

It is unfortunate that the term that we tend to use for such a powerful and important healing phenomenon is the 'placebo effect'. It would be much better and straightforward to call it the 'healing' effect and seek to understand the science of healing better. The administration of placebos smacks of charlatanism, quackery, trickery and is generally seen as intellectually dishonest. This negative connotation is implicit in the origin of the word. In Latin, placebo means, 'I shall please'. It is the first word of the vespers for the dead, which according to Christian liturgy contain verse 9 of Psalm 114 which begins, *'Placebo domino in regione vivorum' (I shall please the Lord in the land of the living).* In the 12th century, these vespers were commonly referred to as placebos, a popular term of derision applied to the incomprehensible nature of these rituals [22]. By the 14th century, the term had become secular and pejorative, suggesting a flatterer or sycophant – a meaning probably derived from the depreciation of the professional mourners, who were paid to sing placebos. So even in the middle ages, the placebo did not have any definitive action but was applied to help the aggrieved cope with their loss and feel better. When the word entered medical terminology, the negative connotation stuck. Placebos were burlesque and counterfeit medicines, often sold at fairgrounds; pills containing dough, sugar and coloured water, whose effectiveness was related entirely to the charisma of the showman.

'I'm O.D. Colognie, the one and only. I've been standing on this bridge since Friday selling Doctor Carter's pink pills for pale people. Guaranteed to purify the blood and make the skin like velvet. Take on an empty stomach and they won't roll off. If the pills don't work, stick the label on the chest and swallow the box.'

Related to the author by his father, Mr Wallace Read

Although most practitioners would be reluctant to acknowledge it, almost all complementary treatments and most of the so called 'active' treatments employed by orthodox medicine probably owe much of their efficacy to the placebo effect. All therapeutic procedures must act at least in part at the level of the idea by inspiring a sense of confidence and belief in their efficacy. Orthodox medicines derived much of their effectiveness because they were prescribed with all the authority of national health institutions and reinforced by medical research. The antibiotics prescribed for colds and sore throats, the antispasmodics for irritable bowels, the vitamin tonics for people who are run down, are difficult to justify on the data derived from controlled clinical trials, but nevertheless they help a lot of people. This is not necessarily bad medicine. Why shouldn't people have treatments that make them feel better? And it is not necessarily dishonest. All of these treatments have some degree of scientific credibility. The prescription of drugs with little or no relevant biological efficacy by doctors and complementary practitioners is not necessarily an intentional deceit. They are usually prescribed in good faith. The doctor believes in them and the patient gets well because he believes in the good faith, backed up by science and authority. This has always been an essential aspect of healing. Indeed, the history of medicine is largely the history of the placebo effect [23].

The insistence of pharmaceutical regulatory authorities on objective evidence has probably undermined the effectiveness of many of the remedies that patients believed in. This may have contributed to a public disillusion with orthodox medicine and led to the increasing popularity of herbal remedies, nutritional supplements and complementary therapies. But now the randomised double blind controlled trials of efficacy, the foundation stone of evidence based medicine, is showing hairline cracks with convincing suggestions that patients can tell from their bodily sensations whether they are receiving the active drug or the placebo. [24]. We should therefore be very cautious lest we sacrifice this essential component of healing on the altar of The National Institute of Clinical Excellence. Instead of trying to restrict the prescription of otherwise useful remedies through the artifice of randomised controlled clinical trials, medical institutions might do better to understand the harness the therapeutic power of the placebo or healing effect.

Placebos are remarkably effective. Roberts and his colleagues have argued that when prescribed with conviction by an enthusiastic practitioner to a patient who has placed his faith in the efficacy of the medication, then response rate is near 100% and the effect can last for years [25]. For example, good or excellent cures of cold sores were reported in 85% patients taking the immunomodulating drug, Levimasole, even though its efficacy was not supported by double blind control trials. The placebo effect can be so convincing that the expected dose ranging effects and the expected unwanted side effects are reported [26].

In therapy and prevention, the idea is as important as the biological effect and in many cases more so. The use of willow bark to treat fevers and aches and pains was a powerful idea since willow grew in swampy areas where fevers and agues were common. The fact that extracts of willow bark also contained aspirin, which has a biological antipyretic and anti-inflammatory effects, not only enhanced its biological efficacy but made it a very effective placebo. Peruvian bark carried the same idea, tinged with a touch of the exotic. It contains quinine. We cannot disconnect placebo effects from biological efficacy. Placebo effects are part and parcel of all biological treatments. The knowledge that a treatment has some biological action, especially if this can be perceived by the patient, gives the treatment 'credibility', and this enhances its therapeutic efficacy. The doctor can prescribe it with conviction and the patient can take it with confidence.

Ian Wickramasekere, Professor of Psychiatry and Behavioural Sciences at Stanford University Medical School has argued that successful therapy requires the appropriate combination of faith and science [21]. Blind faith without reinforcement by science may eventually lead to disillusionment and extinction of the healing effect, while a drug that has an appropriate biological action but is administered without the personal endorsement of the physician can result in a loss of efficacy due to tolerance and habituation. As Rousseau wryly commented as early as 1854, 'You should treat as many patients with the new drugs while they still have the power to heal'.

Credibility is the vital factor in the healing effect. As Christian Xth, King of Sweden, is quoted as saying, '*We console ourselves with our delusions and our imaginings*'. The patient has to believe that the treatment is special, and if the doctor believes it too, so much the better. Voudouris and his colleagues, demonstrated the therapeutic power of belief in an elegant experiment in which an analgesic cream was used to treat the pain induced by applying an electrical current for the forearm [27]. The current was reduced in half of the subjects, giving the impression of greater analgesia. The subjects in whom the current was reduced continued to experience greater analgesic effects of the cream. The placebo works by conditioning, recruiting memories and ideas that are associated with health. Kirsch found that simply calling relaxation therapy, hypnosis, doubled its efficacy in obesity [28]. The propaganda that our diet is unhealthy is etched deep in our unconscious, so redressing the balance with nutritional supplements is a powerful therapeutic idea that must make the people who take supplements a lot better. Nevertheless this therapeutic belief can be influenced by the way it is presented. For example, larger capsules have a greater effect than smaller ones [29], and the enormous and expensive Vitamin C tablets, that are a little larger than a pound coin, are particularly influential. Red pills are said to work better than white for anaemia. Vitamin supplements are usually sold as red or orange capsules. Zinc tablets sold in metallic grey packaging. Evening Primrose Oil is sold in yellow packaging. The packaging is all important because it reinforces the therapeutic belief.

It is not just the proven biological action of the medication that determines the therapeutic efficacy, it is more the way the treatment is given. The most active treatments are rendered useless or are complicated with unwanted side effects if the prescription is tossed across the desk without establishing a sense of connection with the patient. Conversely, sugar pills administered with authority, after eliciting a detailed history and conducting a careful examination, can be remarkably effective [30]. This is the essence of the placebo effect. It harnesses the patients own powers of recovery by implanting the idea of being cared for, inspiring confidence and reducing tension.

A treatment that is concordant with the patients own convictions may well work better for certain conditions than a treatment that has a more potent biological action but which the patient feels uneasy about. That is why so many complementary therapists spend time trying to understand the relationship between the patient and illness and design the treatment to fit the patient, his disease, personality and life experience. This detailed and serious attention to the patient and the design of a special treatment for that patient inspires the faith and confidence that will put the patient on the track to recovery. This is the art of medicine.

Special instructions for when and how the medication is taken enlists the patients involvement in the therapy and helps to reinforce the therapeutic idea. I have found that the anion exchange resin, cholestyramine can be remarkably effective in treating patients with intractable diarrhoea, even when patients say they have taken it before. I explain how bile acids can irritate the colon and cause diarrhoea and how cholestyramine has a special action in binding bile acids. I emphasise to the patient how important it is for them to take the sachet in water 20 minutes before their meals and titrate the dose with the size of the meal. I also encourage them to keep a record of how they have taken the medications so that I can check it the next time I see it.

The way the doctor behaves has an enormous effect on the effectiveness of any prescribed medication. A doctor, who appears calm and confident and exudes a serious air of conviction and authority, pays careful attention to the patient's history, and offers an unhurried explanation of why a particular remedy is likely to be effective, will inspires in the patient a therapeutic feeling of confidence and trust and obtain good responses to treatment. In contrast a busy clinic, a rushed appointment and an exasperated doctor makes the patient feel he has not been listened to, that the doctor does not know what is wrong and does not really care.

Props are important. The consultant's dark suit, the framed medical qualifications, the polished brass plate on the gate, the ordered desk and respectful nurse are traditional artifices that create the impression of confident authority. In contrast, the sloppy-jo jumpers, open neck shirts and 'hush puppies' that so many family doctors wear these days, may create the notion of a friendly neighbour you can talk to over the garden fence but may not exactly inspire confidence. After all, who wants to talk about their piles to the next door neighbour!

The medical consultation can be seen as a piece of theatre, and the skilled exposition of this can dramatically amplify the therapy. Many traditional forms of healing created an atmosphere of authority and awe, that intensified the healing effect. The healing temples of Ancient Greece, the chanting and dances of the African witch doctors, the Red Indian medicine men, the aboriginal healers, conveyed the impression of a special communion with an all powerful spirit world. In the middle ages, all illness was thought to be related to possession by the devil. Only the grave and serious monks in their black habits and towering abbeys had the God given authority and power to exorcise demons.

'A French doctor had a patient who was convinced he was possessed by the devil. The doctor called in a priest and a surgeon, meanwhile equipping himself with a bag containing a live bat. The patient was told it would take a small operation to cure him. The priest offered up a prayer and the surgeon made a slight incision in the man's side. Just as the cut was given, the doctor let the bat fly, crying "behold, the devil is gone." The man believed it and was cured [31].'

Some of the greatest healers in the past were consummate actors and their healing was accompanied by elaborate theatrical preparation. Anton Mesmer used to dress up in a cloak and pointed hat covered in moons and stars and connect his patients to a tub full of iron filings. This created powerful theatre and tapped into the new ideas on electricity and cosmology that were prevalent in the culture. Human disease, like other aspects of human behaviour, is a product of the prevailing cultural ideology [32] and therefore any healing method must tap into the same ideas.

Although few contemporary healers would go as far as Mesmer, the processional ward round of serious white coated healing 'priests' with their unique access, the theatrical conclave in the middle of the ward and the bewildering authority of medical science conveys a similar therapeutic sense of awe and authority. The following contemporary scenario illustrates how effective a simple bit of play acting can be.

'The patient was very demanding and difficult to please and claimed to suffer continuous agony from her ulcer. All of the many mild to moderate analgesics were useless and I did not feel opiates were justified, so I asked the advice of my immediate superior. The superior saw the patient, discussed her pain and with a grave face, said he wanted to try a completely different sort of treatment. She agreed. He disappeared into the office, to reappear a few minutes later, walking slowly down the ward and holding in front of him a pair of tweezers which grasped a large, white tablet. As he came closer, it became clear (to me, at least) that the tablet was none other than effervescent Vitamin C. He dropped the tablet into a glass of water which, of course, bubbled and fizzed, and told the patient to sip the water carefully when the fizzing had subsided. It worked – the new medicine completely abolished her pain' [33].

The doctor was able to ensure the patients positive therapeutic response through his attitude of authority, gravity and seriousness and by providing a special treatment that was so powerful that it fizzed in water and had to be handled with great care.

Injections are more powerful placebos than tablets [34]. Injections of normal saline have cured everything from angina to asthma and from vomiting to vertigo. The analgesic effect of placebos is greater when the patient thinks he is receiving an injection of morphine than other analgesics [26, 35, 36]. Patients in the Villa Maria Roman Catholic mission hospital in Masaka, Uganda, where I worked in 1967, would insist on having a 'Murphy', the injection of coloured saline named after the Irish doctor who had popularised it.

Surgical operations have a greater placebo or healing effect than other forms of treatment. The operating theatre with its gowned and masked players, the quiet atmosphere of concentration and the intimacy of the entry into the patients body conveys an awesome impression. There can be no more powerful an idea than the notion that somebody is going to cut the body open, identify what is wrong and remove the badness. This requires an attitude of paramount authority on the part of the surgeon and one of absolute trust on the part of the patient. In the late 1950s, researchers led by Edmunds G. Dimond of the University of Kansas Medical Centre showed that a sham operation, in which an incision was made on the chest wall was more effective at improving the pain of angina than the then fashionable ligation of the Internal Mammary Artery [37].

Hypnosis is pure theatre, and as well being a powerful therapeutic technique, is a popular form of stage entertainment. Hypnotherapy is the most direct application of the therapeutic power of suggestion and credibility. A trance-like state of relaxed and focussed concentration is induced using techniques of imagery, progressive muscular relaxation and a slow repetitive vocal cadence. This altered state of consciousness renders the patient particularly susceptible to the therapists suggestion. The mental imagery created in hypnotherapists suggestion can create changes in blood flow, [38] brain waves and bowel function. Dr Peter Whorwell uses hypnotherapy to treat The Irritable Bowel Syndrome [39]. He tells his patients to envisage their bowels as a river. If they are constipated he suggests that their river is stagnant and murky and encourages them to change it to a highland stream where the water is clear and tumbling merrily over rocks. I remember applying Whorwell's technique to one of my constipated patients and induced a merry attack of diarrhea that kept the patient confined to home for the next week. The next week I had to slow the stream down to a river gently meandering through meadows and that afforded a more regular bowel habit.

Hypnosis is like the placebo effect without the placebo. Both work by the power of suggestion. Both rely on the patients concentration, expectation and credibility to achieve a therapeutic effect. Hypnosis uses a trance like state to create a powerful mental image. In this respect, it is not unlike the incantations and spells used by traditional healers. The placebo effect, on the other hand, concentrates the imagery around the specific substance or therapy. In this way the medication serves as an amulet, a token or talisman, a lucky charm to ward off the harmful powers that cause the disease. Like the copper bracelets worn by sufferers of rheumatic diseases, the medication is imbued with therapeutic power. Owning it makes the patient feel he is in control of his condition. For many people, the fear of illness induces an attitude of learned helplessness, in which they feel lost and dependant on others. Harold Benson has suggested that if they can have something that allows them to gain control of their illness, then they can replace their learned helplessness by 'remembered wellness' [40]. In this way the locus of control is shifted from the doctor to the patient, who gains in confidence and wellness.

4.3 Who Responds to Placebo Medication

It seems evident that sensitive and vulnerable people of a suggestible disposition that would be more likely to respond better to hypnosis and to placebos. Suggestibility implies a fragile and dependent sense of self that readily attaches itself to external factors to maintain a sense of identity and integrity. The patient puts his faith in the treatment and his imagination and expectation changes the way his body functions and brings about the cure. Robert Burton wrote as early as 1628, 'An empiric oftentimes and a silly chirurgeon, doth more strange cures than a rational physician'... because the patient puts his confidence in him' [41]. And when the commission led by Benjamin Franklin reported to the King of France on the validity of Mesmer's animal magnetism in 1785, they concluded that imagination was the most important factor in explaining the bizarre effects and miraculous cures [42].

It would be mistaken to equate placebo responsiveness with psychopathology; we can all be taken in by a convincing argument. Nevertheless, several authors have observed that patients, who are anxious, dependant and non-critical and those with functional illness respond particularly well to both hypnosis and placebo medication [26, 30, 43].

Following years of careful and detailed observation, Ian Wickramasekere has shown that people who are very susceptible to hypnosis as well as those who are very resistant to hypnosis are prone to functional and psychosomatic disorders and responsive to placebo medication [44]. It is easy to understand how good hypnotic subjects would respond well to placebos. Patients who score highly for hypnotisability are hypersensitive, highly imaginative, empathic, liable to leap from specific experience to general expectations very readily and more likely to experience their feelings to unpredictable factors outside of their control. Such people are said to have porous or permeable psychological 'boundaries'. Events and ideas affect them and may make them feel ill or feel well. It is less easy to understand how subjects who are resistant to hypnosis might also respond well to placebos. Such people are skeptical, rational and analytic and prone to look for mechanical, chemical and physical explanations for their distress. They need to be shown that a particular medication will work. Having experienced benefit, however, they will cling onto the cure as if their life depended on it. These patients respond particularly well to biofeedback techniques in which they can see physiological changes and learn to influence them.

Patients with a brief episode of illness are said to respond better to placebos than those with chronic organic illness. Some patients seem to need to be ill in order to recruit the love and care of their family. They find a sense of purpose and identity in the illness and derive emotional containment from their regular relationship with the family doctor. Such people will respond poorly to any medication, since to be cured will deprive them of the benefits of feeling ill. The patient will continue to take the medication, however, because it validates their identity as an ill person, who needs to be cared for.

It is said that placebos are particularly effective for those conditions that are underpinned by emotional distress [9]. Nevertheless, we all feel vulnerable when we are unwell and we are more likely to exhibit an uncritical acceptance of medicines at those times. Most consumers of nutritional supplements take them, not all the time, but at times of stress, as part of weight reducing regimes, when their spirits are low and when their anxieties are raised by convincing propaganda [45].

4.4 Nutritional Supplements as Placebos

So many people in our society now believe that the food they eat is responsible for their ill health. In a recent study, carried out in our laboratory, 53% of healthy subjects reported food intolerance and most of these identified several putative foods. Among patients with the Irritable Bowel Syndrome, this figure rose to nearly 100%. This belief is heavily reinforced by a sensationalist media. Everyday we receive alarming reports of the risks of food. Red meat and cheese will cause us to get fat, develop high blood pressure and diabetes and die early of heart attacks. The aluminum in our saucepans gives us Alzheimer's Disease. Beef will make us mad and cause colon cancer. Insufficient green vegetables during pregnancy will cause our babies to get hydrocephalus or spina bifida. Too little milk in childhood will cause osteoporosis in later life. Too few antioxidant vitamins or too little fish oil will cause rheumatoid arthritis and coronary artery disease. Such reports fuel the imagination and focus people's insecurities on food. There is now a widespread suspicion that the foods that we eat are contaminated with additives, pesticides, herbicides, and hormones to enhance meat production, or infected with borine spongiform encephalopathy (BSE), salmonella and other microorganisms. People fear that they may make us mad and cause other serious illness. They are suspicious that food is so genetically modified and processed that it is deficient in many of the substances we need to keep healthy. Food is so central to our well-being. Faced with the insistent alarm that the food that we eat is bad for our health, is it surprising that so many people are seeking to protect themselves by taking nutritional supplements? Anything that makes up the deficiencies in our diets or counteracts the toxic substances that we are exposed to must be doing us good. Taking nutritional supplements protect us from illness in much the same way as the invocations, prayers and magic spells protected our ancestors from harm and 'delivered them from evil'.

Nutritional supplements have the necessary credibility to optimise the placebo or healing effect. They offer a logical countermeasure to widespread fears about our diet, they carry the imprimatur of nutritional science, they appear to be endorsed by the medical profession and they are promoted in newspaper articles, television documentaries and advertisements. With the decline of the medical profession as a symbol of authority, people are increasingly influenced by the media. Popular magazines are full of articles advising people how to manage their own health with nutritional supplements or herbal remedies. They suggest daily ingestion of vitamin E or omega-3 fatty acids can reduce the risk of coronary thrombosis, giving vitamin supplements to children can improve IQ, vitamin B_6 can prevent premenstrual tension, and infant deaths can be cut by taking vitamins C and E. A vitamin a day keep the doctor away, especially when presented as coloured capsules, vacuum packed in attractive packages. This is the message many readers of these magazines subscribe to.

We might expect medications that are often taken as prevention or prophylaxis and generate no discernable direct biological change to be subject to extinction or 'placebo sag' [21]. This might well be so if supplements were taken consistently, but the evidence suggests that most people take supplements intermittently when they feel they need them and that they shop around. The market in nutritional supplements and herbal remedies is very volatile. it responds rapidly and vigorously to media scares and the vagaries of fashion. Currently the largest growth area are herbal treatments for sleep and fatigue and pre- and probiotics for gut upsets. In order to maintain sales, companies have to stay ahead of the game, be exquisitely sensitive to media hype and keep creating new indications that alarm and products that soothe a susceptible and vulnerable client base. This can seem to be a cynical exercise in making 'straw men'.

Advertisers and the media are the purveyors of ideas. Advertising has developed into an art form, that permeates our collective consciousness and promotes a familiarity and trust. Through a clever conjunction of ideas, we develop an identification with the product, that makes us want to 'own' it. In television advertising, the product is endorsed by a catch phrase or a tune that serves the same kind of function as the mantra used by mystics and hypnotists to induce a trance like state of suggestibility. This and the fact that people watch television when they are exhausted from the days stresses and sedated with food and alcohol, allows the idea to permeate our imagination and influences the way we think. Television advertising is mini-theatre, the music and the images endorse the idea by tapping into people's emotions, their aspirations, desires, vulnerabilities and fears and the encouraging an identification. In the UK 'size matters' has become a national debate, but has sold a lot of cars. 'Because I'm worth it' is a catch phrase that goes far beyond having shiny hair. The drums, wild horses and breaking waves of the award winning Guinness advert conveyed the image of masculine power barely restrained and coincided with the beer drinking machismo of young men. Just the hint that Vitamin E may make you more potent, that Vitamin B_6 may make you more assertive and confident, that probiotics my protect your children from cancer, creates the anxieties that can only be rectified by the product. Assailed with the sheer sophistication and emotional persuasion of advertising, it not surprising that ill, exhausted, stressed and vulnerable people, worried about the risks of modem living, anxious for the health of their family and desperately looking for something to help them cope, rush to their local pharmacist or health food store and stock up.

4.5 The Ethics of Prescribing or Marketing Placebos as Nutritional Supplements

It is tempting to castigate the prescription of supplements as a deception that severely undermines the trust that must exist between doctor and patient. This situation, however, is not that straightforward. A prescription is only a deception if the doctor is convinced that it has no biological effect but claims that it does. Nutritional supplements are in a kind of hinterland. They are not an inactive treatment. They are essential elements of the diet. Requirements are greater if we are ill and stressed. The fear that modern diets may in some way be deficient in vitamins has received much media coverage. There is a widespread though quite erroneous belief that they cannot do harm. There is also a false assumption that more must be better. Megadoses of vitamin C are sold to help ward off winter colds. This idea has been promoted by a widely respected Nobel laureate, but has been challenged by suggestions that they may enhance the risk of heart disease by thickening arterial walls [46]. Most doctors probably prescribe nutritional supplements in 'good faith'. Even if they are not entirely convinced that they are the most appropriate treatment, vitamins and minerals are essential for life and must therefore do some good. Exhaustion and the pressure of time means that it can be much easier to reach for the prescription pad rather than explain to a patient how their illness may respond better to a change in lifestyle. And more often than not, a patient will expect a prescription and will feel let down and even abandoned if they don't get one. This may lead to an exacerbation of the symptoms.

What is the doctor to do if the patient asserts the conviction that nutritional supplements will help them? Belief and expectation are a major part of the process of healing. Knowing that what the patient believes in is likely to help him, should the doctor disabuse him of that belief. Howard Brody has written that ... 'the physician is not responsible for false beliefs the patient may bring into the encounter, if the physician has taken no action to cause those beliefs'. And when considering the case of a patient with a firmly entrenched belief in the therapeutic powers of vitamins, Brody declares 'that the energetic and prolonged discussion from the physician might mitigate or dispel this false belief, but seems hardly worth the effort given the low probability of harm and the low readiness of the patient to assimilate the new information' [47] But doesn't that just passively encourage trade in 'sham medication? It's a real moral dilemma. If, as I have argued in this article, therapeutic efficacy or healing depends on the unique combination of biological action and belief, then we might conclude that the art of therapy must lie in enhancing the patient's faith in the treatment. But should this justify a blatant deception?

It is very difficult for a doctor to knowingly deceive a patient or to be economic with the truth, even when he realises that a lie would help him more. Ina recent article [30], Mark Chaput de Santoinge and Andrew Herxheimer from The London Hospital have written, 'Attempts to encourage critical thinking towards medical treatment will reduce the placebo effect'. 'Physicians cannot always tell the plain truth'. 'There is a distinction between evasion and deceit'. I am not convinced. The relationship between doctor and patient is a long or – term one and like all such relationships, must be built on trust to be effective. The patient feels weak and insecure and invests a great deal of faith and dependence in his or her doctor. If she discovers that the doctor has lied or been economic with the truth, this can be as bad as the wife who discovers that her husband has cheated. It destroys a bond of trust and like a cancer erodes into the marrow of the relationship undermining all future interactions. How can any relationship work if it is based on deception? 'Freud stressed that the patients insight into the aetiology of his affliction is the one quintessential ingredient that distinguishes the remedial dynamics of his treatment modality from any kind of treatment by suggestion. Treatments by suggestion leave the pathogenic repressions intact and yield only an ephemeral cosmetic prohibition of the symptoms' [48].

In most instances, the dilemma is avoided. Pure placebos are rarely prescribed. The doctor can find some biological justification for the treatment if challenged and the patient knows and trusts this. Credibility is maintained and the patient gets better.

Most nutritional supplements, however, are not prescribed by the doctor but are sold over the counter at pharmacies, supermarkets and health food stores. Surely these cannot be subject to the same ethical debate. After all, if the patient decides to buy nutritional supplements from a shop, then that is a legitimate exercise of his or her free will and should not be subject to any restrictions from a 'nanny state'. It's just the same as buying a car, choosing a holiday or going out for a meal. But is it? We don't necessarily expect a car, a holiday or a meal to make us better or stop us getting ill (although, of course, they may well do). The advertising and sale of nutritional supplements may be seen as the worst form of deception, the implantation of fears into a vulnerable and suggestible population, and the exploitation of these implanted fears for economic gain. Freud thought that setting a fee enhanced the efficacy of the therapy – the patient valued it more and was more committed to it. That's fine if the treatment works, and the patient gets good value for money in terms of the therapist's time and effort. If, on the other hand, it doesn't live up to the 'hype' and the patient has paid good money to get a treatment, the validity of which is dubious, the experience could erode the patients confidence in all other treatments. The making of profit through blatant deception can surely never be justified on ethical grounds. But, manufacturers may argue, 'If there is any deception, the scientists have created it. We cannot judge whether their claims are valid or not. We are making an ethical response to scientific concern and public demand.'

Companies compete in an increasingly cut–throat free market economy. Is it any worse to advertise nutritional supplements to make you feel well, have a better sex life, live longer, look better, be more active, get rid of toxins in the colon than say advertising a hair conditioner than produces that extra bounce or shine. I think there is a world of difference. Nutritional supplements are not cosmetic products, they are consumed as medicines. They act on biochemical processes in the body, they need to be taken in a certain dose and they have toxic effects if taken in excess. They should therefore be subject to the same regulations as drugs. The loophole that treats them as foods and not drugs should be closed with further prevarication. The same principle should apply to herbal remedies. But should we go one stage further? Should the public should be informed if a given supplement has no established efficacy by a notice attached to every advertisement and every packet, like that applied to tobacco advertising? This could be something like, 'This product has no proven efficacy in prolonging life, improving the quality of life or in the treatment of illness'. But if the idea of the treatment has some credibility and makes people feel better and the load on an overburdened health service is reduced, surely undermining credibility with a health warning would be counterproductive.

In some countries, the advertisement of supplements is regulated. For example, the US Food and Drug Administration (FDA) allows companies to state how their products affect the structure or function of the body, but not to make unsubstantiated claims about how they might prevent, treat or cure a disease [49]. That seems a reasonable compromise, but it is hardly likely to make a lot of difference. Patients pick up the idea quickly enough from the images on the advertisements and the media does the rest. Companies are highly dependant on the comment in newspapers, television and the internet. While the company is careful not to make extravagant claims, a hint is enough to encourage the media to do it for them. Publicity can make or break a company in a night and this has little to do with ethics.

Perusing the shelves of my local pharmacist some months ago, I was intrigued to find Mediterranean Diet tablets for sale. There were four choices; Chicory Inulin, Tomato Lycopene, Redwine extract, and Heart Health (containing fish oil). Each costs approximately £6 (10 €) for 28 capsules with the exception of the fish oil capsules which were more expensive. People could cross the road and buy all the ingredients in larger quantities and at a fraction of the cost in the supermarket. A product that is sold under the guise of a currently popular nutritional concept, is cloaked in the mantle of medical and scientific authority. Although the manufacturers did not make any direct claims for the health benefits of their product, there was a heavy implication that you could reduce your risk of cardiac disease to that of Mediterranean countries by taking these supplements. We might be forgiven for thinking that this was an unashamed marketing of an unproven idea, designed to exploit the fears of a vulnerable public. After all it might be that the warmer climate and the outdoor, more sociable Mediterranean life style is more important in reducing cardiac risk than tomatoes, chicory, fish, olives and red wine.

So there's lies, corporate lies, and false statistics. Companies may argue that challenging their sale of supplements would deprive patients of medications which make them feel a lot better. Do we have any right to do that? Doesn't the end justify the means? I do not think it does. We're not talking about deprivation but regulation. Why should companies be allowed to make their profits from a vulnerable population by encouraging a dependency on spurious implications? Instead of frightening and confusing people by conflicting suggestions, surely it is better that the public is clearly informed that the royal road to health involves a moderate, balanced life style – with sufficient attention to rest, exercise, communication, companionship and stress modulation as vital components of emotional health alongside healthy eating and drinking.

4.6 References

1. Euromonitor. Vitamins and dietary supplements. Market research Europe. 31 [Jan-March]. London, Euromonitor Plc. 1999
2. Eisenberg DM, Kessler RC, Foster C, Narlock FE, Calkins DR, Delblanco TL. Unconventional medicine in the United States. Prevalence costs and patterns of use. New England Journal of Medicine 1993; 328: 246–252
3. Ministry of Agriculture Fisheries and Food. National Food Survey, 1997. Annual report on household food consumption and expenditure. London: HMSO, 1998
4. Gregory J, Foster K, Tyler H, Wiseman M. The dietary and nutritional survey of British adults. London: HMSO, 1990
5. Standing Committee on the Scientific Evaluation of Dietary Reference Intakes. Dietary reference intakes for vitamin C, vitamin E, selenium, and beta-carotene, and other carotenoids. The National Academy of Sciences. 2000; 4–7
6. Wickramasekere I. How does biofeedback reduce clinical symptoms and so memories and beliefs have biological consequences? Towards a model of mind-body healing. *Applied Psychophysiology and Biofeedback* 1999; 24: 91–105
7. Kirk SFL, Cade JE, Conner MT, Barrett JH. Supplementary issues for women. Nutrition Bulletin 1998; 23; 197–202
8. Bakal D. Self medication versus self soothing. Minding the body. Clinical uses of somatic awareness. London: The Guildford Press, 2000: 82–129
9. Brown WA. The placebo effect. Scientific American 1998; 278: 90–95

10. Brown GW. Life events and illness. London: The Guilford Press, 1989
11. McEwen BS. Protective and damaging effects of stress mediators. New England Journal of Medicine 1998; 338; 171–179
12. Wessely S, Nimnuan C, Sharpe M. Functional somatic syndromes: one or many? Lancet 1999; 354: 936–939
13. Dunnell K. Are we Healthier? In: Charlton J, Murphy M (eds) *The Health of Adult Britain 1841–1994*. London: The Stationery Office, 1997: 173–181
14. Tofler A. *Future Shock*. London: Pan, 2000
15. Hofer MA. The mother infant interactionas a regulator of infant physiology and behaviour. In: Rosenblum L, Molz H (eds) Symbiosis in parent offspring interactions. New York: Plenum, 1983
16. Wickramasekere I, Wickramasekere IE. A Case Study: Electromyographic correlates in the hypnotic recall of a repressed memory. Dissociation 1997; X[l]: 11–20
17. Stern DN. The First Relationship. Cambridge: Harvard University Press, 1977
18. Winnicott DW. *Transitional objects and transitional phenomena. Through paediatrics to psychoanalysis. Collected papers*. London: Kamac books, 1951: 229–242
19. Brenman E. Hysteria. *International Journal of Psychoanalysis* 1985; 66: 423–432
20. Pearce JMS. The placebo enigma. Quarterly Journal of Medicine 1995; 88: 215–220
21. Wickramasekere I. A conditioned response model of the placebo effect. Predictions from the model. *Biofeedback and Self-Regulation* 1980; 5[l]; 5–14
22. Simini B. Letter. Lancet 1994; 344: 1642–1642
23. Shapiro AK, Morris LA. The placebo effect in medical and psychological therapies. In: Garfield S, Bergin AE (eds) *Handbook of psychotherapy and behavioural change*. New York: Wiley, 2000: 3 69–410
24. Greenberg RP, Fisher S. Examining antidepressant effectiveness. Findings, ambiguities and some vexing puzzles. In: Greenberg RP, Fisher S (eds) The limits of biological treatments for psychological distress. Hillsdale, NJ: Erlbaum, 1989
25. Roberts AH, Kewman DG, Mercier L, Hovell M. The power of non specific effects in healing: implications of psychosocial and biological treatments. Clinical Psychology Review 1993; 13: 375–391
26. Rosensweig P, Brohier S, Zipfield A. The placebo effect in healthy volunteers: influence of experimental conditions on adverse events profile during phase I studies. Clin Pharmacol Ther 1993; 54: 578–583
27. Voudouris NJ, Peck CL, Coleman G. The role of conditioning and verbal expectancy in the placebo response. Pain 1990; 43: 121–128
28. Kirsch 1. Hypnosis as an adjunct to cognitive behavioral psychotherapy: A meta-analysis. Journal of Consulting and Clinical Psychology 1996; 64: 517–519
29. Buckalew LW, Coffield KE. An investigation of drug expectancy, function of capsule colour, size and preparation form. Journal of Clinical Pharmacology 1982; 2: 245–248
30. Chaput de Saintonge DM, Herxheimer A. Harnessing placebo effects in health care. Lancet 1994; 344: 995–998
31. BBC On Line. An anecdote from Denis, Dean of Durham, 1684–1691. Trust Me, I'm a Doctor. 2000
32. Showater E. *Hystories: Hysterical Epidemics and Modem Culture*. London: Picador, 1997
33. Worrall J. Personal communication. In: Grunbaum A (ed) The placebo concept in medicine and psychiatry. Psychological Medicine, 1986: 19–38
34. Blackwell B, Bloomfield SS, Buncher CR. Demonstrations to medical students of placebo responses and non drug factors. Lancet 1972; ii 1279–1282
35. Evans FJ. The placebo response in pain reduction. Advances in Neurology 1974; 4: 289–296
36. Kroenke K, Mangelsdorff D. Common symptoms in ambulatory care: incidence, evaluation, therapy and outcome. Applied Psychophysiology and Biofeedback 1989; 86: 262–266
37. Dimond EC, Kittle CF, Crocket JE. Comparison of internal mammary ligation and sham operation for angina pectoris. *American Journal Cardiology* 1960; 5: 483–486
38. Kopi I. The mechanism of the psychophysiological effects of placebo. Medical Hypotheses 1988; 27: 261–264

39. Whorwell PJ, Prior A, Faraghar EB. Controlled trial of hypnotherapy in the treatment of severe refractory irritable bowel syndrome. Lancet 1984; 2: 1232–1234
40. Benson H, Friedman R. Harnessing the power of the placebo response and calling it remembered wellness. Annals Rev Medicine 1996: 47: 193–199
41. Burton R. The Anatomy of Melancholy. New York: Empire State Book Company, 1628
42. Franklin B. Report of Dr Benjamin Franklin and other commissioners charged by the King of France with the examination of animal magnetism, as now practiced in Paris. London, J. Johnson, 1785
43. Gallimore RG, Turner TL. Contemporary studies of the placebo phenomenon. In: Jewek ME, editor. Psychopathology in the practice of medicine. New York: Appleton Century Crofts, 1978: 51–52
44. Wickramasekere I. Secrets kept from the mind but not the body or behaviour: the unsolved problems of identifying and treating somatisation and psychophysiological disease. Biofeedback and Self-Regulation 1998; 14: 81–132
45. Mintel Marketing Intelligence. Vitamins, minerals and dietary supplements. London: Mintel International Group, Ltd. 1999
46. Ronchetti IT, Quaglino D, Bergamini G. Ascorbic acid and connective tissue. *Subcellular Biochemistry* 1996; 25: 249–264
47. Brody H. The lie that heals. Ann Int Med 1982; 97: 112–118
48. Grunbaum A. *The foundations of psychoanalysis*. A philosophical critique. Berkeley: University of California Press, 1984
49. Gottlieb S. US relaxes its guidelines on herbal supplements. *BMJ* 2000; 320: 208–208

5 Antioxidants, Nutrition and Health

Anthony Diplock

5.1 Introduction

Oxygen derived free radicals are produced within the body's cells by electron transfer reactions usually catalysed by enzymes or transition metal ions, or by ultraviolet or other types of radiation. A free radical may be defined as any species (atom or molecule) capable of independent existence that contains one or more unpaired electrons. An unpaired electron is one that occupies an atomic or molecular orbital by itself and the presence of these unpaired electrons is often associated with increased chemical reactivity, since electrons have an in-built tendency to associate in pairs. Examples of free radicals include the superoxide radical ($O_2^{-}\cdot$) formed in all living cells exposed to oxygen, and the highly reactive hydroxyl radical (OH•), produced from superoxide in the presence of hydrogen peroxide and 'free' (i.e., not protein-bound) transition metal ions.

The production of free radicals is a normal biochemical event. Not all reactions involving radicals are damaging, indeed radicals play a role in many cellular mechanisms. However, if reactive radicals are allowed to come into contact with susceptible biomolecules within cells, this may result in extensive damage, e.g., to DNA, enzymes and other proteins as well as polyunsaturated fatty acids (PUFA) in cell membranes. Extensive cell damage is normally prevented by radical-radical interactions or the action of antioxidants. Deleterious free radical reactions are important in the mechanism of action of some toxins and inflammation and in ischaemia (oxygen deprivation) and reperfusion damage, degenerative arterial diseases, cancer and the ageing process.

5.2 Involvement of Free Radicals in Degenerative Disease and Modulation by Antioxidants

Degenerative diseases such as cancer and cardiovascular disease are multi-factorial processes that take place over a long period of time. Thus for cancer, the well-recognized stages of initiation and promotion lead to a truly transformed cell type; this involves many stages at which free radical involving processes might be implicated; free radical processes may also have a more indirect effect on carcinogenesis. The role of such free radical-involving or -derived processes is of critical importance to the question of whether reduction of risk of cancer by antioxidants is a likely premise. Similarly for cardiovascular disease the process of atherogenesis, which most authorities regard as the precursor to coronary heart disease, certainly involves the formation of oxidised lipid (low density lipoprotein; LDL) at an early stage of the process. This oxidation may be reversed by dietary antioxidants which may thus control the overall process by lowering the rate of oxidation and thus modulate the progress of atherogenesis. The hypothesis is therefore now generally accepted that these two major killer diseases may occur at a slower rate in individuals that have a high level of intake of dietary antioxidants such as vitamins E, C and selenium.

Primary radical species differ markedly in their chemical reactivity, and potential for damage to living cells. Aside from the question of whether it is formed at all in the biological environment, of great potential significance as an initiator of damage is the hydroxyl radical, OH•, since it reacts with most biological macromolecules in its immediate vicinity with rate constants in the order of 10^{-10} or more. This is both an advantage and a disadvantage; the primary damage caused by OH• is likely to be very focal and more probably containable, although it must be appreciated that secondary radicals or radical products may be produced, and that these may be able to move within the intracellular or even intercellular environment, and may be severely detrimental at sites far removed from the point of the initial attack.

5.3 Cancer Aetiology

With respect to damage specifically to DNA, which may be of significance in carcinogenesis, measurement of the production in vivo of modified purine and pyrimidine bases, which are probably derived from DNA excision and repair, has given rise to the estimate that oxygen radicals cause about 10,000 DNA base modifications per cell per day [1]. Such damage by radical species may lead to mutagenesis and carcinogenesis. An account of the effect of free radicals on DNA is that edited by Halliwell and Aruoma [2]. It is clear that damage to DNA may be of primary significance in the aetiology of cancer, by causing direct mutagenic effects, by being involved in the promotion of transformation of mutated cells, as well as in more diffuse effects through expression of genes that may be important in the same context. Both DNA damage and mitogenesis, by agents that increase the rate of mitosis, are thought to be of significance in the cancer process. Four endogenous processes that lead to significant DNA damage are oxidation, methylation, deamination and depurination, and repair mechanisms exist in most cellular systems for these processes [3]. The measurement of DNA adducts has demonstrated that oxidation is likely to be the most significant endogenous damage. Rapidly dividing cells are much more likely to mutate than non-dividing cells and mitogen-induced increases in mitosis expose the cells to greater risk. Lowering the rate of mitogenesis causes a greatly lowered incidence of cancer.

The chemistry of attack by free radicals on DNA is very complex; lesions in chromatin include damage to bases, sugar lesions, DNA-nucleoprotein cross-links. single strand-breaks, and a basic lesions [4]. Hydroxyl radicals, e^-_{aq} and H atoms react with DNA bases by addition and abstraction. Reaction of OH• with both pyrimidines and purines gives several addition products and the detection of specific degradation products of DNA metabolites is probably the best evidence available that OH• formation occurs in vivo. Sugar radicals can be formed by the reaction of OH• with deoxyribose and further reaction of the sugar radicals formed can lead to DNA strand breakage. The further reactions of free radical-altered DNA bases are beyond the scope of this short review. A number of methodologies have been developed for measuring and characterizing these products and the application of these techniques to body fluids offers the possibility of non invasive assessment of free radical damage to DNA in vivo [5]. Detection of altered sugars may also be measured to provide further information about this kind of DNA damage. Singlet oxygen is likely to be involved in these processes. Oxidative modification of guanine and thymine residues, and covalent adduct formation are among the types of reactions that occur. The damage may cause cytotoxicity by block DNA replication which can also give rise to mutation by misreading of modified sites by DNA polymerases or by induction of DNA recombinatorial events; both may be counteracted by the normal cellular repair mechanisms but the possibility exists that, in particular where mitosis is occurring, the repair mechanisms may not be adequate to prevent progression of the damaged cell to a cancerous one.

It is clear that hydroxyl radicals and singlet oxygen produce several different types of damage to DNA, and alkoxyl radicals have also been shown to cause DNA damage [6]. There is however no information available as to the formation of singlet oxygen in the cell nucleus. The reactivity of the oxygen species implies that they must be generated in the nucleus and it is unlikely that migration of such reactive species can account for direct damage to DNA. If it is true that free iron and copper exist in the nucleus [7], then the relatively stable compound hydrogen peroxide, which can migrate freely within cellular structures, may give rise to hydroxyl radicals in situ in the nucleus by Fenton-type reactions. A source of hydrogen peroxide that may be of particular significance in the nutagenic and carcinogenic process is the close proximity of activated phagocytes to the site of initiation of tumorigensis or in sites of inflammation. The oxygen burst associated with the phagocytic function is a considerable source of both hydrogen peroxide and the superoxide anion radical.

An important potential relationship also exists between lipid peroxidation and the causation of mutagenesis and carcinogenesis involving damage to DNA. This is the interaction of aldehyde metabolites of lipid hydroperoxides with DNA which may have consequences for the cell cycle and in carcinogenesis.

There is thus a considerable likelihood that relatively straightforward molecular alterations to DNA structure could lead to mutagenesis and eventual carcinogenesis. However, this is an overly simplistic view and a number of other potential mechanisms of carcinogenesis must also be considered. The involvement of free radicals in cell proliferation has been reviewed by Burdon [8], and the question of the involvement of lipid peroxides and their products in the carcinogenic process has been considered by Cheeseman [9] and by Morrero and Marnett [10]. Lipid peroxides may also affect the rate of cell proliferation through aldehyde products of lipid hydroperoxide breakdown; a variety of carbonyls, such particularly as hydroxyalkenals like 4-hydroxynonenal, may affect enzymic activities and other functions of proteins by their reaction with thiol and amino groups of the protein side-chain. This occurs at high concentrations of the aldehyde and may however have little physiological relevance because of lower concentrations the aldehydes appear to have different effects on cell proliferation, which for example are mediated through effects on adenyl cyclase and phospholipase C activities, and on protooncogene expression which may have considerable significance in the cancer process [8].

The multifactoral nature of carcinogenesis necessitates consideration also of the role of free radicals, and of lipid peroxides in particular, in chemical carcinogenesis. In a review by Morrero and Marnett [10], the metabolic activation of carcinogens by peroxyl radicals is considered and its effect in the metabolic activation of polycyclic hydrocarbons and their DNA conjugates.

5.4 Cardiovascular Disease Aetiology

Coronary artery disease is the chief cause of death in Europe and in the USA. The primary cause of coronary heart disease, and also of stroke and other vascular diseases, is the condition known as atherosclerosis which is characterized by thickening and other pathological degeneration of the arterial intima. It is now thought to be highly likely that the formation of foam cells, which is a very early event in arteriosclerosis, involves oxdative changes in LDL which is capable of being inhibited by the antioxidant nutrients. It is however clear that the events that lead to atherosclerosis are extremely complex and require a detailed knowledge of the biological and biochemical processes involved.

The mechanism of attack by free radicals on polyunsaturated fatty acids is well understood. In arachidonic acid, for example, attack by a radical, such as the hydroxyl radical, abstracts a hydrogen atom from the fatty acid to produce a carbon-centred radical. Following an intermolecular rearrangement which yields a mixture of two products, either the 9- or the 13-carbon-centred radicals, there is attack by these radicals on molecular oxygen which yields either a 9- or a 13-peroxyl radical. These new lipid peroxyl radicals can react with another molecule of unsaturated fatty acid to yield a lipid hydroperoxide and a further lipid radical which will enter the reaction sequence again so that a chain reaction is set up. The chain may be broken by a lipid antioxidant such as α-tocopheroxyl radical. A more detailed description of this reaction sequence is given in [9]. It is presumed that a similar sequence of reactions occurs within the structure of biological membranes, and in LDL within the arterial intima. Spatial constraint of the polyunsaturated fatty acid within the phospholipid in the lipid bilayer lamella structure in membrane may impose constraints on the progress of perioxidation, as well as interception of radicals by membrane proteins with consequent protein damage.

Lipid hydroperoxides are not stable end-products under physiological conditions; they may be exposed to transition metal ions which catalyse the formation of further reactive lipid radical species. In addition there is the possibility that complete degradation of the peroxidized lipid may give rise to products that are biologically active and cytotoxic. Cleavage of carbon-carbon bonds within lipid hydroperoxides formed during perioxidation leads to several different types of product which may be placed in three main classes which are:

(i) Alkanals, typified by malondialdehyde [11], which are highly reactive compounds that can cause considerable intracellular damage by a variety of reactions, which include reaction with protein thiols and cross linking of amino groups of proteins.
(ii) Alkenals, typified in particular by 4-hydroxynonenal (HNE) [12]. The biological activity of these compounds has been explored in some detail and there is no doubt that these compounds are of major significance in cytotoxicity and cytostasis, which are caused by specific effects on the cell cycle. Several reviews of these actions of hydroxyalkenals have appeared [3]. The cytotoxicity of HNE has been demonstrated in a wide range of different cell types [9] but the mechanism of HNE cytotoxicity is not fully understood.
(iii) Alkanes, such as pentane, which is produced as the end product of the oxidation of linoleic and arachidonic acid, and ethane which is derived from linolenic acid [11].

The key role played by low density liporpotein (LDL) oxidation in the early events that lead up to atherogenesis, and the development of coronary heart disease, has become accepted as the principal most likely explanation of a key stage in this complex multifactorial process. The subject has been reviewed in detail [14]. The physical arrangement of the lipids and protein within the LDL particle has been the subject of much study; the particle consists of a central core of cholesterol esters arranged in a lamellar fashion around which cholesterol, phospholipids and apoproteins are distributed. High-affinity receptors for LDL are found on the plasma membrane of most cell types and this receptor is recognized by the apoB_{100} lipoprotein. The primary function of LDL is transport of cholesterol within the body and the function of the receptor is the removal of cholesterol from the circulation, so that it is delivered to extra-hepatic tissues. Since up to 70% of the total cellular receptor activity is located in liver cells, this also provides the mechanism for the return of cholesterol to the liver. The apoprotein of LDL contains ε-lysine modification, is taken up specifically at high rates by macrophage scavenger receptors which differ from the receptors that are responsible for normal LDL metabolism. These scavenger receptors are responsible for the enhanced uptake of cholesterol into macrophages that is observe prior to the formation of foam cells in the atherogenic process. The oxidation of PUFAs within the phospholipids and cholesterol esters of LDL appears to be the first significant process that occurs, and degradation of the resultant lipid hydroperoxides to aldehydic products leads to the formation of Schiff Base complexes with ε-lysine residues within the apoB_{100} lipoprotein. This modification of the LDL apoB_{100} lipoprotein, which occurs within the arterial intima, leads to avid uptake of the oxidized LDL by macrophage scavenger receptors and thus to the beginning of fatty streak formation.

Early studies on the oxidation of LDL in isolated cultured cells demonstrated that the recognition of native LDL by high affinity macrophage receptors was lost and that oxidised LDL (LDL_{ox}) was taken up instead by the scavenger receptors on the macrophage surface. Oxidation of LDL caused oxidation of the PUFAs as indicated above, formation of lysolecithin and a modification of the apolipoprotein B_{100} which involved the loss of available lysine residues that is responsible for the change in receptor specificity, so that the LDL_{ox} was taken up by the scavenger receptors [15]. The suggestion that aldehydes released from the oxidised PUFAs might bind to the ε-amino groups of lysyl residues within the apoprotein has subsequently been confirmed as true. Detailed consideration of the significance and mechanism of LDL oxidation is given in the review [16]. The control of the process of LDL oxidation by vitamin E is central to the role played by LDL oxidation in the aetiology of atherosclerosis and the possible preventive function of the vitamin. Around 30–50% of the plasma vitamin E is located in the LDL fraction, and other antioxidants such as carotenoids are present in much lower amounts. It is therefore reasonable to suggest that the enhancement by dietary means, or by the use of dietary supplements, of LDL vitamin E content could be expected to result in a slowing of the process of LDL oxidation and therefore the arteriosclerotic disease process.

5.5 Reduction of Disease Risk by Antioxidant Nutrients

It is clear from the foregoing that there are many possible ways in which free radical-related events in cellular metabolism may impinge on both the cancer process and the atherosclerotic process in the aetiology of cardiovascular disease. This must provide an excellent rationale, which has not as yet been explained in detail, in which the potential role of antioxidants as agents that reduce the risk of these diseases will eventually emerge. There is however considerable interest in the possibility that dietary vitamin E, vitamin C and β-carotene may be able to lower the risk of a wide range of human diseases. The search for a single protective agent has confused the issue of the link between a high intake of a specified nutrient with lowered risk of a particular disease and the much more extensive evidence that links a high intake of fresh fruit and vegetables with a lower risk.

5.6 Cancer

Reviews of the epidemiological literature have suggested that there is a protective role for vitamin C [17, 18] and β-carotene [19, 20] against the incidence of cancer. In all the studies, where correspondents were asked about fruit and vegetable consumption, it is not certain that the effect that was reported was indeed due to the nutrient in question, and it must be recognized that no allowance was made for the effect of other factors in the foods. Although the evidence linking low intake of any specified antioxidant with elevated risk of cancer is not very impressive there is nevertheless overwhelming evidence that links low incidence of cancer in many body sites with a high intake of fresh fruits and vegetables. In a large meta-analysis of many pieces of evidence [21] this relationship was studied in detail. It was accepted for the purposes of this review that the anticancer activity of carotenoids derives from the action of the carotenoid itself rather than from it first being converted in the body into vitamin A. The methodology of studies in the literature differs somewhat, and the meaning of relative risk, in particular when it is given a numerical value, may differ also. The review used a method by which results can be compared between different studies. Information about intake of a nutrient through diet was obtained by a questionnaire on frequency of consumption of named foods. Respondents were then grouped into those with low, moderate or high intake of individual foods, groups of foods, or of a nutrient contained in them which was calculated. Risk of cancer is expressed as relative risk (RR) and the risk of cancer in the group exposed to a factor (such as low fruit and vegetable intake, or low carotenoid intake) is expressed as a ratio of the risk in the group not so exposed (those with the highest intake). Thus an RR of >1.0 indicates an increased risk of disease, and an RR of 2.0 in a low-consuming group indicates twice the risk of cancer compared with the high-consuming group. Similarly an RR of <1.0 indicates a lowered risk of disease where the same comparison is being made. the statistical significance of the results was based on the results reported by the individual authors: $P<9.95$ or more, the lower level of the 95% confidence interval (CI) at an RR = 1.0. In almost all the studies reviewed adjustment for smoking was made or the effects in smokers were reported separately. There was strong consistency in the data that link a low level of intake of fresh fruits and vegetables with a higher risk of cancer.

At around the time that this work was published, there was a tendency to assume that the effective agents in dietary fruit and vegetables were the antioxidants. This may be far from the true case. Intervention studies that involve specific nutrients have given mixed results. In the study in Linxian in which supplementation with specific vitamin and mineral combinations was undertake [22], it was hoped to reveal whether supplementation with specific vitamins or minerals might lead to lower cancer incidence or mortality. Four combinations of nutrients were tested and doses ranged from one-to two-times the US RDAs. A total of 2127 deaths occurred among trial participants during the intervention period. Cancer was the leading cause of death with 32% of all death being due to oesophageal or gastric cancer. Lower total morality occurred among those subjects receiving supplementation with β-carotene, vitamin E and selenium together (P = 0.03). This reduction was mainly due to lower cancer rates (RR = 0.87, 95% CI = 0.75–1.00) with stomach cancer being especially significant RR = 0.79, (95% CI = 0.64–0.99), with the reduction in the risk being apparent 1–2 years after the supplementation began.

The Finnish α-Tocopherol β-Carotene (ATBC) study of 29,133 heavy chronic smokers tested the effects of 20 mg β-carotene, either alone or in combination with 50 IU vitamin E for an average of 6 years. There was a significant increase of lung cancer incidence (16%) in the groups which received β-carotene [23]. A more detailed analysis of the results revealed that the increased risk of lung cancer appeared to be restricted to participants who had smoked more than 20 cigarettes per day over an average period of 30 years [24].

The β-Carotene and Retinol Efficacy Trail (CARET) of 18,914 subjects at high risk for lung cancer (heavy smokers, and asbestos-exposed workers) evaluated that combination of 30 mg β-carotene and 25,000 IU vitamin A over an average of 4 years. The intervention group had a significantly increased risk of lung cancer (RR = 1.36 [25]. A reduced risk of lung cancer (RR = 0.800 was seen in subjects who were former smokers at the beginning of the study. interestingly, participants with high initial serum β-carotene concentrations had a 31% reduction in risk of lung cancer (P = 0.03), regardless of which group they were randomized to. This effect was also seen in the ATBC study and Physicians' Health Study which was conducted over 12 years in 22,071 male physicians who consumed 50 mg β-carotene every second day. there was no beneficial influence of β-carotene on cancer incidence. However due to the long duration of the trail, it is important to note that there were no adverse effects reported.

Mixed messages emerge at present from the literature concerning intervention with individual antioxidants in the cancer process. A major factor that contributes to this confusion is undoubtedly the timing of the intervention; in both the ATBC and CARET studies, intervention was made following many years of high risk behaviour, smoking, at a time when it would be expected that many of the subjects would have been in a pre-cancerous condition. It is clear that the intervention was apparently instrumental in turning this precancerous state in some individuals into overt cancer, and the explanation for this is not immediately apparent. However it nevertheless seems likely that intervention with β-carotene at a much earlier stage of the cancer process would have been more likely to have had beneficial results, because it is particularly at those early stages that free radicals are thought to have their major impact.

If it becomes likely that an increase in the human dietary intake of antioxidants is to be recommended as a means designed to lower the risk of cancer, then it must be certain that this proposal will be without risk due to some toxic effect. With respect to vitamin C, the conclusion from an exhaustive survey of the literature is that oral intake of high (up to 200 mg/day) have not been consistently reported to result in side effects although some reports of low reliability may suggest that minor side-effects may occur. With regard to vitamin E the following conclusions which were reached [26, 27] with respect to the safety of oral intake of vitamin E by human subjects, and are endorsed here. (i) The toxicity of vitamin E is very low. (ii) Animal studies show vitamin E is not mutagenic, carcinogenic or teratogenic. (iii) Reported increases in serum lipids in human subjects following high oral dosage are inconsistent and of little significance. (iv) In double blind human studies, oral dosage resulted in few side-effects, even at a dosage as high as 3.2 g per day. (v) Dosage up to 100 mg per day is considered to be entirely safe and without side-effects. (vi) Oral intake of high levels of vitamin E can exacerbate the blood coagulation effect of vitamin K deficiency: high vitamin E intake is contra-indicated in these subjects. With regard to β-carotene, supplementation of normal individuals in the population with moderate supplements can be undertaken safely.

5.7 Cardiovascular Disease

A confounding factor in studying the relationship between vitamin E and cardiovascular disease is the variation in the blood triglyceride and cholesterol levels of patients with heart disease. Changes in vitamin E levels needed to be judged against the background of changes in the level of triglyceride and cholesterol. Thus it was found [28] that, when fasting blood samples from 116 healthy volunteers were analysed for vitamin E and blood lipids, there was a strong association between vitamin E and the serum lipid concentrations in those who did not smoke but that the rise in the serum level in a cohort of smokers was not associated with a corresponding rise in vitamin E level. Similarly [29] when vitamin E, cholesterol and triglycerides were measured in sera from 167 patients with angina pectoris. An increase in the concentration of vitamin E was observed only in patients with lipidaemia, where as the vitamin E content was similar to that of a control population in patients with hypertension, in smokers and in patients free of hyperlipidaemia. A correlation was found between vitamin E and triglyceride level of the samples ($r^2 = 0.52$). These data also correspond to data from another part of the study in which 224 men and 435 women without ischaemic heart disease were examined. In the men, vitamin E content was found to be correlated with triglycerides ($r^2 = 0.50$) and in the women with cholesterol. The ratio of vitamin E to triglyeride level is thus a more reliable index of vitamin E status in human subjects. It was concluded [30] that 'the plasma status of topcopherol can conclusively be interpreted only in comparison to the level of plasma lipids' and he introduced the term 'lipid-standardized vitamin E' which was used to indicate the degree of saturation of plasma lipids by vitamin E which may be taken as the only reliable index of the vitamin E status of an individual. This measure which is in line with advice offered by Horwitt some years earlier [31], has been adopted and used consistently by workers in the field since that time.

Many aspects of the antioxidant hypothesis for disease prevention were brought together for the first time [30] when the available evidence was discussed that showed an association between high intake of antiodidant nutrients and low incidence of ischaemic heart disease; the following points were made. (i) The accumulation of lipid hydroperoxides within arteriosclerotic plaque correlated with the extent of arteriosclerosis, which highlights the possibility that oxidation of lipid might be a primary event in plaque formation. (ii) Peroxidised diets in many cases lead to toxicity expressed through degenerative heart disease in animals. (iii) Peroxidised low density lipoprotein is cytotoxic to endothelial cells in culture. (iv) Endothelial or smooth muscle cells in culture could generate lipid peroxidation products that could modify apoprotein B of LDL. (v) Experimental myocardial necrosis induced by catecholamines, hyperbaric oxygen or by ischaemia and subsequent reperfusion, is accompanied by lipid peroxidation, inhibited by antioxidants. (vi) Plasma of patients with ischaemic heart disease contains elevated levels of thiobarbituric acid reacting substances. (vii) Marginal deficiency of vitamin E in animals caused functional and morphological alterations in heart muscle and arterial walls.

Data from the pilot WHO/MONICA study [30] showed some inverse correlation, in particular with respect to vitamin C and vitamin E, between the medians of the plasma parameters measured and incidence of coronary heart disease mortality. The main WHO/MONICA study was designed to monitor (hence MONI-) determinants of cardiovascular (hence –CA) disease in 39 collaborating centres in 26 European countries [32]. In the Vitamin Substudy statistical medians of the plasma antioxidant levels in approximately 100 randomly assigned apparently healthy males (40–49 yrs of age) selected at each of 16 study sites were measured and correlated with the established age-specific ischaemic heart disease mortality for men who were 40–59 years of age; the mortality figure used was the established mean value for at least the preceding three years. The ischaemic heart disease differed six-to seven-fold between the lowest as compared to the highest mortality figures [33] and the methodology is described in detail, including particularly the technique of lipid standardization of the levels of vitamin E to common concentrations of cholesterol (5.7 mmol/l) and triglycerides (1.25 mmol/l). The classical risk factors, total plasma cholesterol, blood pressure and smoking habits, did not reveal correlations in univariate analysis with ischaemic heart disease mortality risk which itself differed within the twelve groups by six-to seven-fold although there were some variations in the classical risk factors within a small band of normal values and for cholesterol the variation was 5.1–6.2 mmol/l. This is an important observation because it enabled study of the relationship between blood antixiodant levels in these 12 study populations, and the risk of ischaemic heart disease without the need to allow for confounding effects caused by variation in plasma cholesterol level which is regarded as classical risk factor. Where it was found that classical risk factors were comparable for all the groups examined, there was a statistically significant inverse correlation ($P = 0.002$) between the age-specific ischaemic heart disease mortality and the absolute unadjusted, plasma level of vitamin E which in univariate analysis gave the strong correlation of $r^2 = 0.63$. Lipid standardization of the plasma vitamin E levels improved the significance of the inverse relationship with mortality so that the correlation coefficient was now $r^2 = 0.73$. Four study populations were found to have plasma cholesterol levels that lay outside the band of values (5.1–6.2 mmol/l) that was chosen for the 12 population subgroup; two of these, from Finland, lay above the chosen band and two, from Italy lay below it. When these study populations with high or low blood cholesterol levels were included using lipid standardization vitamin E levels, there was also a statistically significant inverse correlation and the correlation coefficient was $r^2 = 0.62$.

Edinburgh, in Scotland has been identified as a city with a high incidence of ischaemic heart disease (298/100,000; n = 108) [33]. To test the hypothesis that plasma concentrations of antioxidant nutrients might be related to the risk of angina, and to measure the extent to which such risk is independent of classic risk factors for coronary heart disease, a study was conducted [34]. In this case-control study a sample of 6,000 men aged 35–54 was surveyed by a postal questionnaire. To avoid the confounding effect of dietary changes in subjects who had been diagnosed as having heart disease and had been advised by their doctor to make dietary changes, only subjects who had had chest paid and had never seen a doctor were included in the study. The 125 angina cases who were identified were compared with 430 healthy subjects without any symptoms of heart disease and complete data were obtained for 110 angina cases and 394 control subjects. Measurements of plasma vitamins and non-fasting lipids, and platelet fatty acid composition, was made at once without storage of the samples; adipose tissue was sampled under local anaesthetic. There was found to be a statistically significant ($P<0.01$) difference between the controls and the cases with respect to smoking habit (respectively 29% and 46%); no other classical risk factors were found to be of significance including plasma total and HDL cholesterol. There was no significant difference between the vitamin A and unadjusted vitamin E levels, and there was a significantly lower level of carotene ($P<0.001$), vitamin C ($P<0.01$) and lipid adjusted vitamin E ($P<0.01$) in the plasma of the angina cases. In this population case-control study, low plasma concentrations of vitamin E, vitamin C and β-carotene were found to be related to an increased risk of angina pectoris in men. For plasma vitamin E the relationship remained significant after adjustment for age, blood pressure, total and HDL cholesterol, non-fasting triglycerides, relative weight and smoking status and it was concluded that some populations with a high incidence of coronary heart disease might benefit by increasing their intake of antioxidant nutrients, particularly vitamin E.

The results of the Health Professionals Study (The Physician's Study) and the Nurses' Health Study, were published in 1993 [35, 36]. The Physician's Study is a prospective investigation of 51,529 male health professionals who were aged 40–75 years in 1986 when the study began. A number of the subjects were excluded for dietary or health reasons, and the remaining 39910 men were eligible for inclusion in the follow-up study. The 1986 questionnaire enquired about frequency of intake of 131 foods and ten additional questions specifically addressed the current use of vitamin supplements. Case assessment was from records of fatal coronary disease, non-fatal, myocardial infarction, coronary artery bypass grafting and percutaneous transluminal coronary angioplasty. Each participant's follow-up time began with the date of the 1986 questionnaire and continued until the diagnosis of an end-point, death or January 1990 whichever came first. Relative risks were calculated by dividing the incidence rate of coronary disease among the men in each category of antioxidant intake by the rate for the men in the lowest category of disease. For the age-adjusted and multivariate relative risk of coronary heart disease according to quintile group for the intake of vitamin E, as compared to the men in the lowest quintile group for vitamin E, men in the highest quintile group and an age-adjusted risk of coronary disease of 0.59 (95% CI, 0.47–0.7; $P<0.001$). The total intake was further subgrouped according to dietary or supplemental sources. The maximal reduction in risk is shown in men who consumed 100–400 IU/day with no further increased reduction at higher doses of E. There was also found to be a suggestion of an inverse trend between duration of use of vitamin E and the risk of disease. Men who reported use of vitamin E supplements for 10 or more years had a relative risk of 0.65 (95% CI 0.46–0.92) compared to non-users. The multivariate relative risk of coronary heart disease among men taking specific vitamin E supplements (i.e. not multivitamin supplements) was 0.75 (95% CI 0.61–0.93) as compared with non-users. Among men who took vitamin E supplements in doses of at least 100 IU/day for two or more years the relative risk was 0.63 (95% CI 0.47–0.84). The reduction in relative risk of coronary artery disease associated with the highest quintile group for total vitamin E intake was slightly less among current smokers (RR 0.67, 95% CI 0.34–1.31) compared to those who had never smoked (RR 0.52, 95% CI 0.34–0.78).

The Nurses' Health Study [36] began in 1976 with 121,700 female registered nurses. A total of 87,245 women remained in the study following the usual exclusions. Similar criteria and questionnaires as those used in the men's study (see above) were employed to obtain information as to possible relationships between vitamin E intake and the relative risk of coronary heart disease. During 679,485 person-years of follow-up from 1980 to 1988, 552 cases of major coronary heart disease were identified and documented. There was a statistically significant reduction in risk of coronary disease among women with a high intake of vitamin E compared to those with a low intake. Adjustments for age and smoking history showed clearly that the lower risk of heart disease was primarily associated with taking a vitamin E supplement. In a multivariate model that controlled for a number of risk factors, the relative risk associated with the use of specific vitamin E supplements was 0.61 (CI 0.45–0.81) and this was improved further by excluding users of less than 100 IU of vitamin E per day for less than two years (RR = 0.52, 95% CI 0.34–0.89).

A study in Finnish men [37] found that the titre autoantbodies to oxidatively modified LDL was a predictor of the progression of carotid atherosclerosis. Antibodies against epitopes of oxidised LDL had previously been shown to recognize material in atherosclerotic lesions in rabbit and in man [38–40]. In the study of [37] the titre was measured of autoantibodies to malondialdehyde (MDA)-modified LDL (MDA-LDL), in baseline serum samples from 30 Eastern Finnish men with accelerated two year progression of carotid atherosclerosis and 30 age-matched controls. The men with high atherosclerotic score had a significantly higher titre of MDA-LDL (P = 0.003). Cases also had a higher proportion of smokers (37% vs 3%), higher LDL cholesterol (4.2 mmol/l vs 3.6 mmol/l) and a higher serum copper concentration.

A more recent intervention study shows a clear effect of vitamin E on the reduction of angiographically proven coronary atherosclerosis [37a]. Patients (2002) were enrolled following rigorous screening as to their suitability and followed up for a median of 510 days; 1035 were given 800 IU R,R,R,-α-tocopherol for the first 546 patients and 400 IU for the remainder, 976 patients received placebos. The primary endpoints were a combination of cardiovascular death and non-fatal myocardial infarction (MI), as well as non-fatal MI alone. The plasma α-tocopherol levels were found to show a considerable rise in the treated groups, but did not change in the placebo groups. α-Tocopherol treatment significantly reduced the risk of the primary trial endpoint of cardiovascular death and non-fatal MI (41 vs 64 events; RR 0.53, 95% CL 0.34–0.83, P = 0.005), which was due to the reduction in risk of non-fatal MI (14 vs 41 events; RR 0.23, 95% CL 0.11–0.37, P = 0.005). There was however a non-significant excess of cardiovascular deaths in the α-tocopherol-treated group (27 vs 23 events). The conclusion was that in patients with angiographically proven symptomatic coronary atherosclerosis, α-tocopherol treatment substantially reduced the rate of non-fatal MI, with beneficial effects apparent after 1 year of treatment. This study raises a number of questions as to the mechanism of the beneficial effect of vitamin E; some authors have commented that it may have been due to a reduction of coronary atherosclerotic lesions; others have suggested that the mechanism may be mediated through thrombotic effects and alteration in blood platelet function.

The evidence reviewed here makes a compelling case for the likelihood that the risk of cardiovascular disease may be lowered by increasing the intake in human populations of vitamin E. Taken together with the biochemical rationale which has been advanced for the mechanism of atherosclerosis there is a very compelling case for the possibility that vitamin E may have a direct preventive function in the development of atherosclerosis and subsequent coronary disease, as well as perhaps having some therapeutic effect in patients with established heart disease. With respect to the epidemiological evidence it is particularly striking that low incidence of cardiovascular disease is negatively correlated with vitamin E levels in three kinds of study. Thus, in the MONICA/WHO cross-cultural comparison of 16 European study populations [41], in the case-control study of angina pectoris [34], and in the very large Health Professionals' Studies which were in the nature of intervention trials although the intervention with vitamin E was self-determined [35, 36], vitamin E was consistently associated with lowered risk of disease. It must however be stressed that epidemiological data cannot establish causal relationships and can only point to relationships which must be tested by other means. It remains therefore a matter of judgement to decide whether the relationship is likely to be a causal one, as Steinberg points out in his excellent Editorial [42], and 'that judgment will be affected by the strength of the relationship, its consistency, its biological plausibility and other criteria'.

5.8 References

1. Ames BN, Shingenaga MK, Park EM. In: Davies KJA, editor. Oxidation Damage and Repair: Chemical, Biological and Medical Aspects. New York: Pergamon; 1991. pp 181–187
2. Halliwell B, Aruoma OI. DNA and Free Radicals. 1st ed. New York, London: Ellis Horwood; 1993
3. Ames BN, Shigenaga MK. Oxidants are a major contributor to cancer and aging. In: Haliwell B, Aruoma OI, editors. DNA and Free Radicals. New York and London: Ellis Horwood; 1993. pp 1–15
4. Dizdaroglou M. Chemistry of free radical damage to DNA and nucleoproteins. In: Halliwell B, Aruoma OI, editors. DNA and Free Radicals. New York and London: Ellis Horwood; 1994. pp 19–39
5. Halliwell B. Oxidative DNA damage: meaning and measurement. In: Halliwell B, Aruoma OI, editors. DNA and Free Radicals. New York and London: Ellis Harwood; 1993
6. Meneghini R, Martins EL. Hydrogen peroxide and DA damage. In: Halliwell B, Aruoma OI, editors. DNA and Free Radicals. New York and London: Ellis Horwood; 1993. pp 83–93
7. Thorsten K, Romslo I. Uptake of iron from transferring by isolated hepatocytes. Biochim Biophys acta 1984; 804: 200–208

8. Burdon R Free radicals and cell proliferation. In: Rice-Evans CA, Burdon RH, editors. Free Radical Damage and Its Control. Amsterdam, London, New York and Tokyo: Elsevier; 1994. pp 153–183
9. Cheeseman KH. Lipid peroxidation and cancer. In: Halliwell B, Aruoma OI, editors. DNA and Free Radicals. New York and London: Ellis Horwood; 1993. pp 109–144
10. Merrero R, Marnett LJ. The role of organic peroxyl radicals in carcinogenesis. In: Halliwell B, Aruoma OI, editors. DNA and Free Radicals, New York and London: Ellis Horwood; 1993. pp 145–61
11. Tappel AL, Dillard CJ. In vivo lipid peroxidation: measurement via exhaled pentane and protection by vitamin E. Fedn Proc 1981; 40: 174–178
12. Esterbauer H. Lipid peroxidation products Formation chemical properties and biological activities. Free Radicals in liver injury 1985: 29–47
13. Esterbauer H, Koller E, Heckenast P, Moser R, Celotto C. Cytotoxic lipid peroxidation products. First Vienna Shock forum 19877: 24–52
14. Rice-Evans C, Bruckdorfer KR. Free radicals, lipoproteins and cardiovascular dysfunction. Molec Aspects Med 1992; 13: 1–111
15. Steinbrecher UP. Oxidation of human low density lipoprotein results in derivitisation of lysine residues of apolipoprotein B by lipid peroxidation decomposition products. J Biol Chem 1987; 262: 3603–3608
16. FrucHart JC, Duriez P. Free radicals and atherosclerosis. In: Rice-Evans CA, Burdon RH, editors. Free Radical Damage and Its Control. Amsterdam, London, New York and Tokyo: Elsevier, 1944. pp 253–76
17. Block G, Menkes M. Ascorbic acid in cancer prevention. In: Moon TE, Micozzi MS, editors. Diet and cancer prevention: investigating the role of micronutrients. New York: Marcel Dekker 1989. pp 341–388
18. Block G. Vitamin C and cancer prevention: the epidemiologic evidence. Am J Clin Nutr 1991; 53: 270S–282S
19. Ziegler RG. A review of epidemiologic evidence that carotenoids reduce the risk of cancer. J Nutr 1989; 119: 116–122
20. Basu TK, Temple NJ, Hodgson AM. Vitamin A, β-carotene and cancer. Prog Clin Biol Res 1988; 259: 255–267
21. Block G, Patterson B, Subar A. Fruit vegetables and cancer prevention: a review of the epidemiological evidence. Nutr Cancer 1992; 18: 1–29
22. Blot WJ, Li JY, Taylor PR, Guo W, Dawsey S, Wang GQ et al. Nutrition intervention trials in Linxian, China: Supplementation with specific vitamin-mineral combinations, cancer incidence and disease-specific mortality in the general population. J Nat Cancer Inst 1993; 85: 1483–1492
23. ATBC*. The effect of vitamin E and β-carotene on the incidence of lung cancer and other cancers in male smokers. New Engl J Med 1994; 330: 1029–1035
24. Albanes D, Heinonen OP, Taylor PR, Virtamo J, Edwards BK, Rautalahti M et al. α-Tocopherol and β-carotene supplements and lung cancer incidence in the α-tocopherol, β-carotene prevention study: effects of base-line characteristics and study compliance. Journal of the National Cancer Institute 1996; 88(21): 1560–1570
25. Omenn GS, Goodman GE, Thornquist MD, Balmes J, Cullen MR, Glass A et al. Effects of combination of β-carotene and vitamin A on lung cancer and cardiovascular disease. New Engl J Med 1996; 334: 1150–1155
26. Kappus H, Diplock AT. Tolerance and safety of vitamin E: a toxicological position report. Free Rad Biol Med 1992; 1391): 55–74
27. Diplock AT. Safety of antioxidant vitamins and β-carotene. American Journal of Clinical Nutrition 1995; 62(6 Suppl): 1510S–1516
28. Ellis NI, Lloyd B, Lloyd RS, Clayton BE. Selenium and vitamin E in relation to risk factors for coronary heart disease. J Clin Pathol 1984; 37(2): 200–206
29. Cherniauskene R, Margiavichene LE, Varshkiavichene ZZ, Gribauskas PS. (Vitamin E and serum lipids in ischemic heart disease). Vopr Med Khim 1984; 30(3): 102–105

30. Gey KF. On the antioxidant hypothesis with regard to arteriosclerosis. *Biblthca Nutrit dieta* 1986; 37: 53–91
31. Horwitt MK, Harvey CC, Dahm CH, Searcy MT. Relationship between tocopherol and serum lipid levels for determination of nutritional adequacy. Annals of the New York Academy of Sciences 1972; 203: 223–236
32. WHO. World Health Organisation. The WHO MONICA Project. World Health Stat Q 1989; 42: 27–149
33. Gey KF, Puska P, Jordan P, Moser UK. Inverse correlation between plasma vitamin E and mortality from ischemic heart disease in cross-cultural epidemiology. Am J Clin Nutr 1991; 53: 326S–34S
34. Riemersma RA, Wood DA, Macintyre CC, Elton RA, Gey KF, Oliver MF. Risk of angina pectoris and plasma concentrations of vitamins A, C and E and carotene. Lancet 1991; 337(8732: 1–5
35. Rimm EB, Stampfer MJ, Ascherio A, Giovannucci E, Colditz GA, Willett WC, Vitamin E consumption and the risk of coronary heart disease in men. N Engl J Med 1993; 328(20): 1450–1456
36. Stampfer MJ, Hennekens CH, Manson JE, Colditz GA, Rosner B, Willett WC. Vitamin E consumption and the risk of coronary disease in women. N Engl J Med 1993; 328(20): 1444–1449
37. Saonen JT, Yla-Herttuala S, Yamamoto R, Butler S, Korpela H, Salonen R et al. Autoantibody against oxidised LDL and progression of carotid atherosclerosis. The Lancet 1992; 339: 883–888
37a. Stephens NG, Parsons A, Schofield PM, Kelly F, Cheesman K Michinson MJ. Randomised controlled trial of vitamin E in patients with coronary disease: Cambridge Heart Antioxidant Study (CHAOS). Lancet 1996; 347: 781–786
38. Haberland ME, Fong D, Cheng L. Malondialdehyde-altered protein occurs in atheroma of Watanabe heritable hyperlipidaemic rabbits. Science 1988; 241: 215–218
39. Boyd HC, Gown AM, Wolfbauer G, Chait A. Direct evidence for a protein recognized by a monoclonal antibody against oxidatively modified LDL in atherosclerotic lesions from a Watanbe heritable hyperlipidaemic rabbit. Amer J Pathol 1989; 135: 815–825
40. Palinski W, Rosenfeld Me, yla-Herrtuala S. Low density lipoprotein undergoes oxidative modification in vivo. Proc Natl Acad Sci USA 1989; 86: 1372–1376
41. Gey KF, Moser UK, Jordan P, Stahelin HB, Eicholzer M, Ludin E. Increased risk of cardiovascular disease at suboptimal plasma concentrations of essential antioxidants: an epidemiological update with special attention to carotene and vitamin C. Am J Clin Nutr 1993; 57: 787S–97S
42. Steinberg B. Antioxidant vitamins and coronary heart disease [editorial; comment]. N Engl J Med 1993; 328(20): 1487–1489

6 Nutritional and Non-Nutritional Uses of Vitamin B_6

David A. Bender

6.1 Introduction

Nutritional deficiency of vitamin B_6 is essentially unknown, although a significant proportion of the population in developed countries show biochemical evidence of inadequate or marginal vitamin B_6 nutritional status, despite intakes that meet or exceed reference intakes, suggesting that current estimates of requirements may be too low. Furthermore, since estimates of requirement are based on prevention of deficiency, it is relevant to consider whether somewhat higher intakes may be beneficial in terms of promoting optimum nutrition.

Vitamin B_6 has been used to treat a wide variety of conditions, which may or may not be related to inadequate intake. In some conditions use of vitamin B_6 supplements has been purely empirical; in other conditions there is a reasonable physiological or metabolic mechanism to explain why supplements of the vitamin many times greater than average requirements may have therapeutic uses. However, even in such conditions there is little evidence of efficacy from properly conducted controlled trials.

At high levels of intake (in excess of 100 mg/day, compared with reference intakes of 1.5–2 mg/day) vitamin B_6 is neurotoxic, and there have been reports of (partially reversible) sensory nerve damage among people taking supplements of 1000 mg/day.

In June 1997 the UK Department of Health Committee on Toxicity [1] proposed limits on the amounts of vitamin B_6 that may be supplied in supplements. The proposals can be interpreted as an attempt to differentiate between levels of intake that may be considered to be nutritionally relevant and higher levels that can be considered to be for pharmaceutical purposes, to treat a disease or condition:

- up to 10 mg may be sold freely as a nutritional supplement (this is some 6-fold higher than the reference intake, although the figure was derived by extrapolation from toxicological data);
- 10–50 mg/day may only be sold in a pharmacy, where professional advice is assumed to be available;
- over 50 mg/day may only be provided on prescription, since at or above this level of intake there is considered to be a risk of adverse effects, which therefore have to be balanced against the benefits in treating a clinical condition.

The proposals generated very considerable controversy, with arguments both from those who opposed all regulation of nutritional supplements and those who did not oppose regulation, but questioned the scientific evidence on which the limits had been established. In July 1998 the proposed legislation was put in abeyance, pending further examination of the evidence concerning toxicity of the vitamin. This chapter aims to provide an overview of the requirements for vitamin B_6, a summary of the evidence for the pharmacological uses of vitamin B_6 and finally a discussion of drug interactions and toxicity of vitamin B_6.

6.2 Metabolism and Metabolic Functions of Vitamin B_6

Six vitamers have vitamin B_6 metabolic activity: pyridoxine, pyridoxal and pyridoxamine, and their 5′-phosphates (see Fig. 1). The metabolically active coenzyme is pyridoxal 5′-phosphate. In the liver there is rapid oxidation of the other vitamers to pyridoxal, and rapid phosphorylation to pyridoxal phosphate, which is the main circulating vitamer, exported from the liver bound to albumin. Uptake into peripheral tissues is by extracellular dephosphorylation, followed by metabolic trapping inside the cell as pyridoxal phosphate. Pyridoxal phosphate that is not bound to enzymes is rapidly dephosphorylated, and surplus pyridoxal in tissues is oxidised to pyridoxic acid, which is the main urinary metabolite of the vitamin [2].

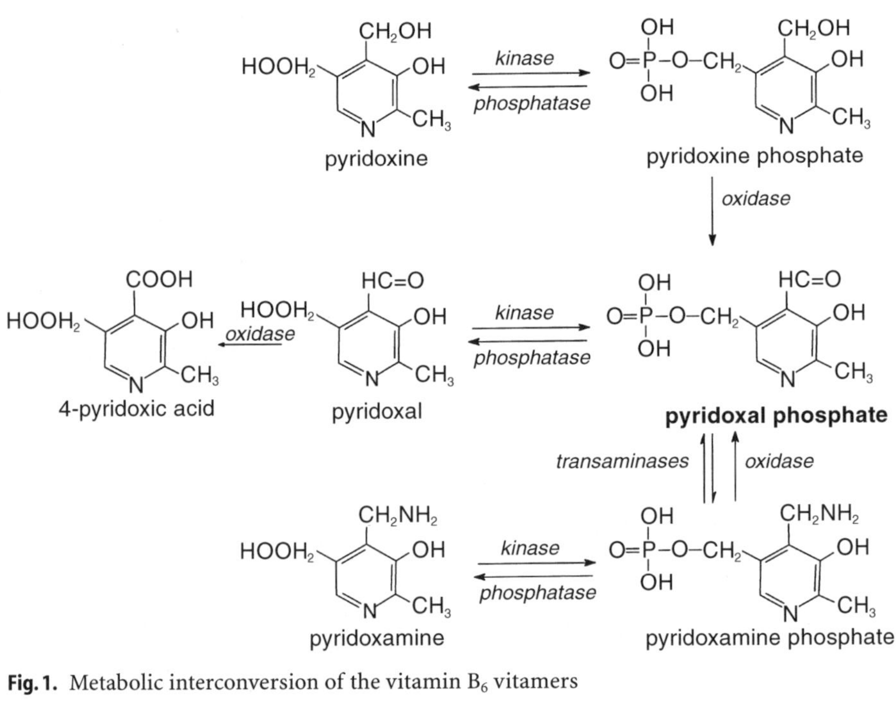

Fig. 1. Metabolic interconversion of the vitamin B_6 vitamers

Vitamin B_6 has activities in three main areas: as a coenzyme in amino acid metabolism, as the coenzyme of glycogen phosphorylase, and in regulation of the activity of steroid hormones on target tissues.

In amino acid metabolism the aldehyde group of pyridoxal phosphate reacts with the ε-amino group of the substrate; reactions of pyridoxal phosphate-dependent enzymes include:

a) transamination of amino acids to yield their keto-acids (oxo-acids), which are then oxidised as metabolic fuels. The reverse reaction is also important for the synthesis of non-essential amino acids from keto-acids that are common metabolic intermediates, such as oxaloacetate, ketoglutarate, pyruvate, etc;
b) decarboxylation of amino acids to yield amines, which are neurotransmitters or hormones, such as γ-aminobutyrate (GABA), histamine, noradrenaline (and hence adrenaline), serotonin;
c) a variety of reactions involving the side-chains of amino acids, including kynureninase (EC 3.7.1.3) in tryptophan metabolism, and cystathionine synthase (EC 4.2.1.22) and cystathionase (EC 4.4.1.1) in methionine and homocysteine metabolism;
d) decarboxylation of phosphatidylserine to phosphatidylethanolamine in phospholipid synthesis.

In glycogen phosphorylase pyridoxal phosphate acts as a phosphate buffer at the active site of the enzyme. Before this catalytic rôle was established, it was assumed that muscle acted as a storage pool of vitamin B_6; some 70–80% of total body vitamin B_6 is in muscle associated with this enzyme. However, pyridoxal phosphate is not released from muscle in depletion or deficiency, although it is released in prolonged fasting, when glycogen reserves are depleted, and there is an increased requirement for pyridoxal phosphate in the liver for transamination of amino acids for gluconeogenesis.

Pyridoxal phosphate also acts to terminate the actions of steroid and other nuclear-acting hormones, including vitamins A and D and thyroid hormone. It binds to a lysine residue in the hormone receptor protein, displacing it from binding to the hormone-response element on DNA, and so ending the enhancement of gene expression. Studies in experimental animals have shown that various steroid hormones are accumulated in the nucleus of target tissues to a greater extent, and for longer, in vitamin B_6 deficiency, with some evidence of enhanced end-organ responsiveness to low doses of hormones. Studies with cells in culture have shown that acute vitamin B_6 depletion (achieved by addition of the antimetabolite 4-deoxypyridoxine) leads to a two-fold increase in hormone-stimulated rate of expression of expression of genes with a variety of hormone-response elements, and conversely, addition of high concentrations of pyridoxal to the culture medium results in a halving of the rate of gene expression in response to the hormones [3, 4].

6.3 Requirements and Reference Nutrient Intakes

Clinical deficiency of vitamin B_6 is more or less unknown; the only reported cases were in the early 1950s, associated with infant milk formula that had been severely overheated in manufacture, leading to the formation of pyridoxyllysine by reaction between the aldehyde group of the vitamin and the ε-amino groups of lysine in protein. Not only is pyridoxyllysine nutritionally unavailable as a source of the vitamin, but it also has antivitamin activity [5].

Estimates of requirements from which reference nutrient intakes (RNI) are derived are based on studies in which subjects were fed controlled diets deficient in vitamin B_6, then, after the development of metabolic abnormalities were repleted with graded levels of intake – i.e. depletion/repletion studies. The criterion of adequacy in such studies is normalisation of one or more of the following biochemical indices of status during repletion:

a) excretion of xanthurenic and kynurenic acids after a test dose of tryptophan (the tryptophan load test, see Fig. 3);
b) excretion of homocysteine after a test dose of methionine (the methionine load test, see Fig. 2);

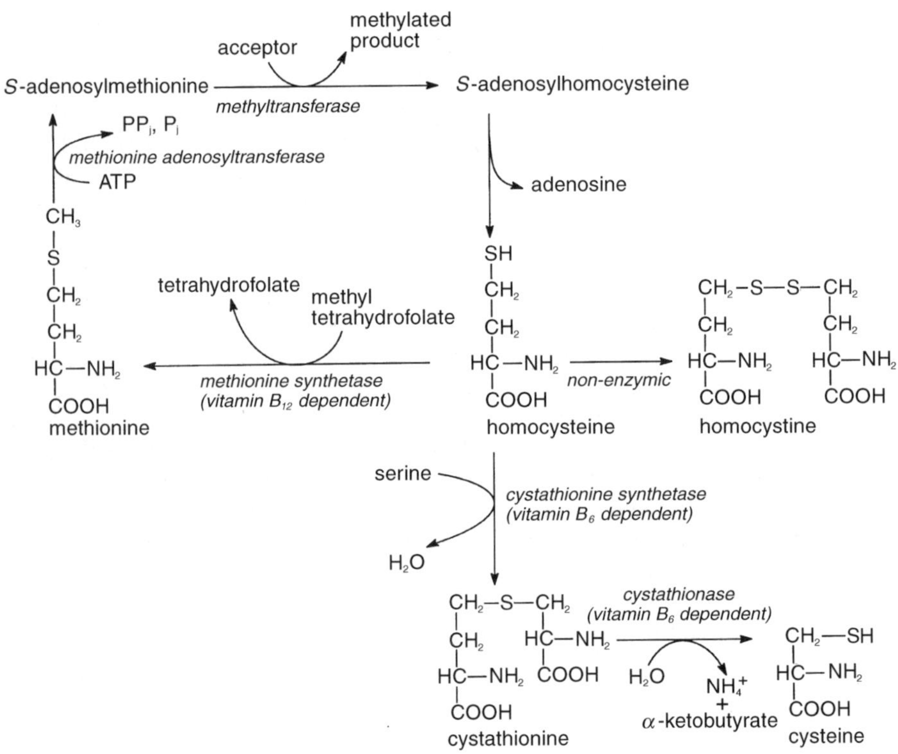

Fig. 2. Homocysteine and methionine metabolism

c) plasma concentration of pyridoxal phosphate or total vitamin B_6;
d) urinary excretion of 4-pyridoxic acid;
e) activation of red cell aspartate or alanine apo-transaminase by pyridoxal phosphate added in vitro – the transaminase activation coefficient.

Although some 70–80% of total body vitamin B_6 is associated with muscle glycogen phosphorylase, and is not involved in amino acid and protein metabolism, this pool has a slow turnover; the remaining 20–30% of the body pool, which is largely associated with amino acid metabolism, has a more rapid turnover. It is therefore likely that protein intake, or the burden of amino acids to be metabolised, will have a significant effect on vitamin B_6 requirements. Certainly the depletion/repletion studies demonstrated that biochemical evidence of depletion developed more rapidly during depletion in subjects fed a high protein diet, while repletion required a higher intake of the vitamin, than in subjects fed a low protein diet.

Current reference intakes in most countries are calculated on the basis of 15 or 16 μg vitamin B_6/g dietary protein intake. For average intakes of protein this leads to an RNI of 1.4–1.6 mg/day for adults. More recent studies suggest that the requirement to meet the most sensitive criteria of adequacy in depletion/repletion studies in women indicate a RNI of 20 μg/g protein. It is not clear whether this represents a gender difference (most of the earlier studies were performed on men) or whether the more recent studies were more sensitive in detecting marginal inadequacy [6–8].

Average intakes in most countries are significantly above reference intakes. However, a number of studies have reported that 10–20% of adults show biochemical evidence of inadequate vitamin B_6 nutrition by one or other of the two criteria most commonly used: plasma concentration of pyridoxal phosphate or erythrocyte transaminase activation coefficient. This suggests that current estimates of vitamin B_6 requirements may be too low, although there is little evidence that marginal plasma concentrations of pyridoxal phosphate or marginally elevated transaminase activation coefficients have any functional significance [8].

6.4 Potential Benefits of Higher Levels of Intake: Homocysteine Metabolism

The identification of hyperhomocysteinaemia as an independent risk factor in atherosclerosis and coronary heart disease [9] has led to suggestions that intakes of vitamin B_6 higher than are currently considered adequate to meet requirements may be desirable. Homocysteine is intermediate in methionine metabolism, and may undergo one of two metabolic fates, as shown in Fig. 2: remethylation to methionine (a reaction that is dependent on vitamin B_{12} and folic acid), or onward metabolism leading to the synthesis of cysteine (trans-sulphuration). Therefore intakes of folate, vitamin B_{12} and/or vitamin B_6 may affect homocysteine metabolism.

The trans-sulphuration pathway has two pyridoxal phosphate dependent enzymes: cystathionine synthetase and cystathionase, and in vitamin B_6 deficiency there is disturbance of methionine metabolism, with development of hyperhomocystinaemia and homocystinuria. This provides the basis of the methionine load test for vitamin B_6 status.

Epidemiological studies suggest that hyperhomocysteinaemia is most significantly correlated with low folate status, but there is also a significant association with low vitamin B_6 status [10]. Results from the Nurses' Health Study in the USA [11] show that cardiovascular disease risk is lowest among those women with the highest intakes of folate and vitamin B_6. Since the sources of both vitamins for those people with the highest intakes were fortified breakfast cereals and multivitamin supplements, it is not possible to distinguish between any potential protective effects of the two vitamins.

Trials of supplementation have shown that while folate supplements lower fasting homocysteine in moderately hyperhomocysteinaemic subjects, supplements of 10 mg/day vitamin B_6 have no effect [12–14]. In one series of studies [13, 14], vitamin B_6 supplements reduced the peak plasma concentration of homocysteine following a test dose of methionine. This can probably be explained on the basis of the kinetics of the enzymes involved; the K_m of cystathionine synthetase is 10-fold higher than that of methionine synthetase. Under basal conditions, little homocysteine is metabolised by way of the trans-sulphuration pathway; it is only after a loading dose of methionine, when homocysteine rises to high levels, that the activity of cystathionine synthetase, rather than the concentration of its substrate, is limiting.

It thus seems unlikely that intakes of vitamin B_6 above amounts that are adequate to prevent metabolic signs of deficiency will be beneficial in lowering plasma concentrations of homocysteine [15].

6.5 Pharmacological Uses of Vitamin B_6

A number of (very rare) genetic conditions are known in which a pyridoxal phosphate dependent enzyme has a defect in the coenzyme binding site, and only has significant activity when the tissue concentration of pyridoxal phosphate is very much higher than normal. Affected children can be maintained in normal health by providing supplements of 200–1000 mg vitamin B_6/day throughout life [16]. These vitamin B_6 dependency syndromes conditions include:

a) convulsions of the newborn due lack of γ-aminobutyrate (GABA) as a result of a defect in glutamate decarboxylase;
b) cystathioninuria due to a defect in cystathionase (see Fig. 2);
c) gyrate atrophy with ornithinuria, due to a defect in ornithine-δ-aminotransferase;
d) a variant of homocystinuria, due to a defect in cystathionine synthetase (see Fig. 2);
e) a variant of primary hyperoxaluria, type I, due to a defect in peroxisomal alanine glyoxalate aminotransferase;
f) sideroblastic anaemia due to a defect in δ-aminolevulinate synthetase and hence decreased haem synthesis;
g) xanthurenic aciduria due to a defect in kynureninase (see Fig. 3).

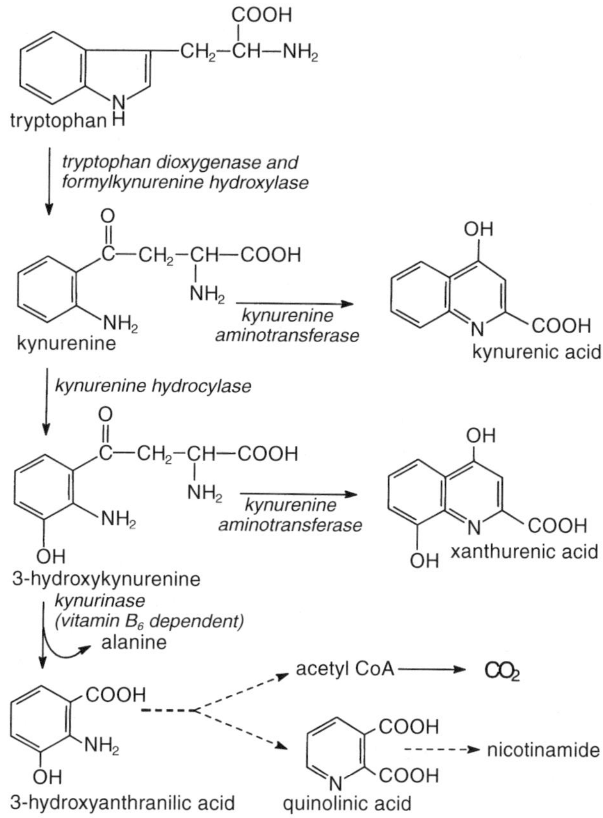

Fig. 3. The oxidative pathway of tryptophan metabolism

Supplements of vitamin B_6 ranging from 25–500 mg/day have been recommended for treatment of a variety of conditions, discussed below, in which there is an underlying physiological or biochemical mechanism to justify their use, although in most cases there is little evidence of efficacy. It has also been used empirically, with little or no evidence of efficacy, in the treatment of a variety of conditions including: acute alcohol intoxication, atopic dermatitis, autism, dental caries, diabetic peripheral neuropathy, Down's syndrome, Huntington's chorea, schizophrenia, and steroid dependent asthma.

Some reports have shown vitamin B_6 to be effective in suppression of lactation, although others have shown no difference from placebo. Because the vitamin suppresses the increase in prolactin induced by treatment with the dopamine receptor antagonist pimozide, and because lactation is also suppressed by the dopamine agonist bromocriptine, it has been suggested that it acts to stimulate dopaminergic activity in the hypothalamus. However, it is more likely that its action is by reduction in target tissue responsiveness to the steroid hormones that stimulate prolactin secretion [17].

6.5.1 Side-Effects of Oral Contraceptives

The high-dose oral contraceptives of the 1960s had a variety of side effects, including depression of mood and impaired glucose tolerance. A number of studies showed that supplements of 100 mg/day vitamin B_6 relieved the depression and normalised glucose tolerance in women taking these contraceptives. More recent studies have shown that the side effects of low-dose combined oral contraceptives (nausea, vomiting, dizziness, depression and irritability) show no better response to 150 mg vitamin B_6/day than to placebo [3].

Apparent vitamin B_6 deficiency in women taking high-dose oestrogen-progestagen contraceptives was first reported by Rose in 1966 [18]. He reported impaired metabolism of tryptophan, with increased urinary excretion of xanthurenic and kynurenic acids after a test dose of the amino acid (see Fig. 3). Since then there have been many reports of abnormal tryptophan metabolism in women taking both oral contraceptives and menopausal hormone replacement therapy, which have generally been interpreted as indicating oestrogen-induced vitamin B_6 deficiency or depletion.

In many cases tryptophan metabolism has been normalised by supplements of 20–50 mg of vitamin B_6/day, but not by nutritionally relevant amounts. Furthermore, when indices of vitamin B_6 status other than tryptophan metabolism have been assessed (e.g. the metabolism of a test dose of methionine, plasma concentrations of B_6 vitamers or the activation of erythrocyte transaminases by pyridoxal phosphate added in vitro), these have been normal, suggesting that the impairment of tryptophan metabolism may be due to an effect other than vitamin B_6 depletion [3].

One explanation of the beneficial effect of vitamin B_6 supplements on tryptophan metabolism in women taking oestrogens, and indeed of the extreme sensitivity of tryptophan metabolism as an index of vitamin B_6 status, may lie in the enzymology of kynureninase. In common with a number of other pyridoxal phosphate dependent enzymes, kynureninase catalyses, slowly, the half-reaction of transamination as an alternative to its usual reaction. This results in formation of pyridoxamine phosphate at the active site of the enzyme, and loss of activity. The enzyme can only be reactivated if there is a sufficiently high concentration of pyridoxal phosphate to displace pyridoxamine from the catalytic site and reform the active holo-enzyme. Normally there is a considerable amount of catalytically inactive kynureninase in the liver, which is activated by addition of pyridoxal phosphate in vitro; this may be either true apo-enzyme or enzyme that has been inactivated by transamination [19].

Another factor which may account for the reduction in excretion of tryptophan metabolites after a test dose in people receiving relatively high supplements of vitamin B_6 is the effect of pyridoxal phosphate on enzyme induction by steroid hormones. The rate of entry of tryptophan into the oxidative pathway is limited by the activity of tryptophan dioxygenase, which is induced by glucocorticoid hormones; high intakes of vitamin B_6 would be expected to reduce synthesis of the enzyme by terminating hormone action, so reducing metabolic flux through the pathway.

It was noted above that there is little evidence that oestrogens cause vitamin B_6 deficiency or depletion, and although the metabolism of a test dose of tryptophan is abnormal, other indices of vitamin B_6 status are not. Oestrogen metabolites are competitive inhibitors of kynureninase, and will impair tryptophan metabolism, leading to results of a tryptophan load test similar to those seen in vitamin B_6 deficiency, but by a completely different mechanism. This suggests that the tryptophan load test is not a useful index of vitamin B_6 status for use in field studies, although it is still useful in experimental depletion/repletion studies to determine requirements [20].

6.5.2 Impaired Glucose Tolerance and Diabetes Mellitus

Some 18% of women taking high dose oestrogen oral contraceptives showed impaired glucose tolerance, which return to normal on withdrawal of the steroids [21]. Impaired glucose tolerance is also common in pregnancy, and may be severe enough to be classified as diabetes mellitus – so-called gestational diabetes, which usually resolves on parturition. Both in women taking these oral contraceptives, and in gestational diabetes, a number of studies have shown that supplements of around 100 mg of vitamin B_6/day result in improved glucose tolerance [22]. However, other studies have shown that while vitamin B_6 supplements normalise tryptophan metabolism in pregnancy, they do not improve glucose tolerance.

There are derangements of tryptophan metabolism in pregnancy, which resemble those seen in vitamin B_6 deficiency. As discussed above, oestrogen metabolites inhibit kynureninase, and they also lead to reduced activity of kynurenine hydroxylase (EC 3.7.1.3) and hydroxyanthranilate oxidase (EC 1.10.3.5), although the mechanisms involved are unclear [23]. In experimental animals, pregnancy has effects on tryptophan metabolism that are additive to those seen in vitamin B_6 deficiency, and are resistant to modest supplements of the vitamin. As a result, in pregnancy or in response to (high dose) oral contraceptives, tissue concentrations of kynurenine, hydroxykynurenine and xanthurenic and kynurenic acids are higher than normal.

The impairment of glucose tolerance associated with high plasma levels of oestrogens may be due to a high plasma concentration of xanthurenic acid, which forms a biologically inactive complex with insulin [24]. The improvement following high doses of vitamin B_6 could then be explained by activation of apo-kynureninase or reactivation of kynureninase that has been inactivated as a result of transamination. However, animal studies have failed to demonstrate any effect of xanthurenic acid administration on glucose tolerance, and it has been suggested that the improvement in glucose tolerance in response to vitamin B_6 was due to increased formation of quinolinic acid as a result of relief of the impairment of kynureninase activity [25]. Quinolinic acid is an inhibitor of phosphoenolpyruvate carboxykinase, one of the key enzymes of gluconeogenesis, and the administration of tryptophan, to increase synthesis of quinolinic acid, has also been reported to improve glucose tolerance.

There are conflicting results on the effects of vitamin B_6 status on glucose tolerance other than impairment associated with pregnancy or use of high-dose contraceptives. There seems to be no effect of marginal vitamin B_6 status on glucose tolerance or insulin secretion in response to a glucose load in people with non-insulin dependent diabetes. Indeed, there is one report that in a group of non-diabetic subjects with marginal vitamin B_6 status glucose tolerance was in fact better than in those with adequate status [26]. The response of plasma insulin to the glucose load was normal, suggesting enhanced sensitivity to the hypoglycaemic action of insulin in marginal vitamin B_6 deficiency. Other studies have reported that in isolated pancreatic islets from vitamin B_6 deficient rats there is impaired secretion of insulin, and plasma insulin is significantly lower than normal in the deficient rats in response to a glucose load [27, 28].

There is some evidence that pyridoxal phosphate may be beneficial in overcoming some of the effects of poor glycaemic control in diabetes. In vitro pyridoxal phosphate inhibits the non-enzymic reaction between lysine and glucose (the Maillard reaction). Administration of pyridoxal phosphate to genetically diabetic mice has been reported to reduce the thickening of the glomerular basement membrane, which has been attributed to non-enzymic glycation of connective tissue proteins [29]. In one study of men with non-insulin dependent diabetes [30], supplements of 150 mg vitamin B_6/day led to a significant reduction in glycated haemoglobin, and hence improved oxygen transport capacity, although there was no change in glycaemic control. While these results suggest beneficial effects of vitamin B_6 supplementation in diabetes, the reduced glycation of proteins is due to reaction between pyridoxal phosphate and the amino groups that would otherwise be glycated.

Overall there is little convincing evidence either that vitamin B_6 supplements will be of any use in the treatment of diabetes (possibly apart from gestational diabetes), nor that vitamin B_6 deficiency is a significant factor in the development of diabetes.

6.5.3 Depression

There is a great deal of evidence that deficiency of serotonin (5-hydroxytryptamine) or the catecholamines (dopamine, noradrenaline and adrenaline) is a factor in depressive illness, and many antidepressant drugs act to decrease the catabolism of amines or enhance their interaction with receptors. A key enzyme involved in the synthesis of serotonin and the catecholamines is aromatic amino acid decarboxylase (EC 4.1.1.28), which is pyridoxal phosphate dependent. Therefore, it has been suggested that vitamin B_6 deficiency may result in reduced formation of the neurotransmitters, and so be a factor in the aetiology of depression. Conversely, it has been suggested that supplements of vitamin B_6 may increase aromatic amino acid decarboxylase activity, and so increase amine synthesis and have a mood elevating or antidepressant effect.

There is little evidence that vitamin B_6 deficiency affects the activity of aromatic amino acid decarboxylase [31]. In patients with kidney failure, undergoing renal dialysis, the brain concentration of pyridoxal phosphate falls to about 50% of normal, with no effect on serotonin, catecholamines or their metabolites [32]. However, like kynureninase, aromatic amino acid decarboxylase can undergo self-inactivation by catalysing transamination, and it is possible that at times of low availability of pyridoxal phosphate, reactivation of the enzyme may be impaired, so that supplements of vitamin B_6 may have an antidepressant action by increasing serotonin synthesis.

In rats, high doses of vitamin B_6 (10 mg/kg body weight) lead to decreased oxidative metabolism of tryptophan, an increased plasma concentration of tryptophan, and increased uptake of tryptophan into the brain, leading to an increased rate of serotonin turnover [33]. This suggests that vitamin B_6 supplements might be a useful adjunct to tryptophan for the treatment of depression. It is likely that the impairment of tryptophan oxidation is the result of reduced induction of tryptophan dioxygenase by glucocorticoid hormones in the presence of high concentrations of pyridoxal phosphate.

Overall, however, there is little or no evidence from clinical trials that vitamin B_6 is effective in the treatment of depressive illness.

6.5.4
The Premenstrual Syndrome

The studies showing that vitamin B_6 supplements were effective in overcoming some of the side effects of (high dose) oral contraceptives have led to the use of vitamin B_6 in treatment of the premenstrual syndrome – the condition of nervousness, irritability, emotional disturbance, headache and/or depression suffered by many women for up to 10 days before menstruation. There is no evidence that women who suffer from premenstrual syndrome have any lower vitamin B_6 status that do others, and the doses used have been in the region of 50–200 mg/day, which is very much higher than would be required to correct any deficiency of the vitamin [34–36].

Twelve placebo-controlled double-blind trials of vitamin B_6 in the premenstrual syndrome have been reviewed by Kleijnen et al. [37]; the evidence of beneficial effects is weak. In three of the studies there was a significant beneficial effect of vitamin B_6 supplements of 100, 300 or 500 mg/day. Supplements of 50 mg/day were reported to have a significant beneficial effect on depression, irritability and tiredness, but none of the other premenstrual syndromes. Supplements of 150 mg/day led to some improvement in dizziness, vomiting and behavioural changes, but considerable physical and affective symptoms remained. Five studies yielded ambiguous results, and a further three reported: an improvement for 82% of subjects receiving 100 mg vitamin B_6/day, and 70% of those receiving placebo; a positive trend but no statistical significance using 200 mg/day; and disappointing and 'not clear' results using 50 mg/day. The remaining four studies reported no beneficial effects of doses between 100–500 mg/day.

Interestingly, one study [38] which reported no significant difference between vitamin B_6 (100 mg/day) and placebo, showed that whichever treatment was used second in a double-blind cross-over trial was significantly better than the treatment used first.

Despite the lack of evidence of efficacy, the major use of vitamin B_6 supplements, either prescribed or self-prescribed, is in the treatment of premenstrual syndrome.

6.5.5
Morning Sickness

Doses of vitamin B_6 between 50–200 mg have an anti-emetic effect, and the vitamin has been used to overcome the nausea associated with radiotherapy. It has also been used, empirically, since the 1940s to treat morning sickness in pregnancy. It was included together with doxylamine succinate in Bendectin (Debendox), which was prescribed for treatment of morning sickness, and later withdrawn on suspicion of teratogenicity. There is little or no evidence of teratogenic effects of the combined formulation, although the effects of vitamin B_6 on responsiveness to steroids and retinoids might affect critical stages on embryological development [39].

There is no evidence that women who suffer from severe nausea and vomiting in pregnancy have any lower vitamin B_6 nutritional status than others. Two studies give some evidence of efficacy. A double blind trial of vitamin B_6 (25 mg every 8 hours for 3 days) led to a significant reduction in vomiting, and an improvement in nausea in those who initially reported severe nausea [40]. By contrast, in a trial of 30 mg/day for 5 days there was a significant decrease in nausea, with a non-significant trend indicating a reduction in vomiting [41]. Several workers have noted that as morning sickness is a self-limiting condition, it is difficult to perform well-controlled trials.

6.5.6
Carpal Tunnel Syndrome

Carpal tunnel syndrome (compression of the median nerve as it passes through the carpal tunnel, the space between the bones of the wrist and the connective tissue over the flexor tendons) is a major source of occupational health problems. A number of studies have suggested that inadequate vitamin B_6 status is an aetiological factor or that supplements may relieve the condition, although there is no physiological reason to expect vitamin B_6 to have any effect on the aetiology or progression of the condition.

The early work in this area, and indeed most of the reports of a beneficial effect of vitamin B_6, have come from one group of workers [42, 43]. These studies suggest that vitamin B_6 deficiency, as assessed by erythrocyte aspartate aminotransferase activity, is associated with carpal tunnel syndrome, and responds only slowly to administration of doses of 100–200 mg of vitamin B_6/day for up to 12 weeks.

A review of a number of studies [44] concluded that vitamin B_6 deficiency was unlikely to be associated with occupational carpal tunnel syndrome, and noted that all studies published at that time were flawed by a lack of scientific design.

In a double-blind controlled study [45] vitamin B_6 had no advantage over placebo or no treatment at all; in a randomised prospective trial of vitamin B_6 or placebo, there were no differences in electrophysiological signs, clinical signs or symptoms between the two groups.

It thus appears that while there is some suggestion of symptomatic relief in open trials, there is no evidence from double-blind placebo controlled trials that vitamin B_6 is effective in treating carpal tunnel syndrome.

6.5.7 Hypertension

Vitamin B_6 depletion leads to the development of hypertension in experimental animals, which is normalised within 24 hours by repletion with the vitamin. Four mechanisms, which are not mutually exclusive, have been proposed to account for this [46]:

a) Central effects on blood pressure regulation as a result of decreased synthesis of brain γ-aminobutyric acid (GABA) and serotonin (5-hydroxytryptamine). Glutamate decarboxylase activity in the nervous system is especially sensitive to vitamin B_6 depletion, possibly as a result of mechanism-dependent inactivation by transamination. While there is no evidence that aromatic amino acid decarboxylase activity is reduced in vitamin B_6 deficiency, there is reduced formation of serotonin in the central nervous system [47].
b) Increased sympathetic nervous system activity. There is evidence of elevated plasma concentrations of adrenaline and noradrenaline in vitamin B_6 deficient animals [48].
c) Increased uptake of calcium by arterial smooth muscle, leading to increased muscle tone, and hence increased circulatory resistance and blood pressure. This could reflect increased sensitivity of vascular smooth muscle to calcitriol (vitamin D) action in vitamin B_6 deficiency; the membrane calcium-binding protein is regulated by vitamin D and vascular tissue has calcitriol receptors [49].
d) Increased end-organ responsiveness to glucocorticoids, mineralocorticoids and aldosterone. Over-secretion of (and presumably also enhanced sensitivity to) any of these hormones can result in hypertension. Vitamin B_6 supplementation would be expected to reduce end-organ sensitivity to these hormones, and thus might have a hypotensive action.

A number of studies suggest that supplements of vitamin B_6 may have a hypotensive action. Supplements of 300 mg vitamin B_6/kg body weight/day attenuated the hypertensive response of rats treated with deoxycorticosterone acetate [50]. At a more realistic level of supplementation (five times the usual amount provided in the diet) vitamin B_6 prevented the development of hypertension in the Zucker *(fa/fa)* obese rat. Withdrawal of the vitamin supplement led to the development of hypertension [51]. In patients with essential hypertension, supplements of 5 mg/kg body weight/day led to reduced blood pressure [52].

6.6 Drug Interactions with Vitamin B_6

The antituberculosis drug isoniazid (*iso*-nicotinic acid hydrazide) reacts non-enzymically with pyridoxal phosphate to form a metabolically inactive hydrazone, resulting in functional vitamin B_6 deficiency [53]. This is most commonly seen as secondary pellagra, due to impaired activity of kynureninase (see Fig. 3), and hence impaired synthesis of nicotinamide nucleotides from tryptophan. The pellagra responds to supplements of vitamin B_6. Isoniazid also leads to the development of peripheral neuropathy, which responds to vitamin B_6 supplements. This has led to the belief that vitamin B_6 deficiency causes peripheral neuropathy, although there is no evidence of this. The neuropathy seems to be an effect of isoniazid intoxication; the response to vitamin B_6 is the result of removing isoniazid as the pyridoxal adduct, rather than repleting vitamin B_6 deficient tissues [54].

When relatively high doses of isoniazid were used to treat tuberculosis, it was common to give vitamin B_6 supplements – this had no effect on the therapeutic action of the drug, but did prevent the peripheral neuropathy and secondary pellagra. When lower doses of isoniazid were introduced, in a therapeutic cocktail with other medication, vitamin B_6 supplementation became less usual. However, cases of isoniazid-induced pellagra have been reported among people taking low doses of isoniazid; it is likely that many of those affected were genetically slow acetylators of isoniazid, so that a low dose was, for them, equivalent to a higher dose for a fast acetylator [55]. There have been a number of reports of successful treatment of acute isoniazid intoxication with vitamin B_6 supplements.

Other hydrazine derivatives can also cause vitamin B_6 depletion by forming hydrazones, leading to the development of secondary pellagra, including the anti-Parkinsonian drugs Benserazide (Roche) and Carbidopa (Merck, Sharp and Dohme) [56].

When dopa was first introduced for the treatment of Parkinsonism, one of the most frequent side effects was persistent nausea and vomiting. Because of the (slight) evidence that vitamin B_6 has an anti-emetic and anti-nauseant action, supplements were given together with dopa. The result was a considerable reduction in the efficacy of dopa in controlling Parkinsonian signs and symptoms; the magnitude of the effect was related to the dose of pyridoxine given. The problem was due to the formation of a stable adduct between pyridoxal phosphate and dopa, which not only reduced the concentration of dopa available for uptake into the brain, but also acted as an inhibitor of aromatic amino acid decarboxylase [57].

Theophylline therapy for asthma can cause seizures, apparently as a result of reaction with pyridoxal phosphate, leading to low plasma concentrations, and hence reduced synthesis of GABA in the central nervous system. The administration of vitamin B_6 to mice treated with theophylline reduces the number of seizures; in rabbits, vitamin B_6 reverses the changes in electro-encephalogram caused by high doses of theophylline [58].

High doses of vitamin B_6 may lower blood concentrations of anticonvulsant medication such as phenytoin and phenobarbitone, apparently by increasing the rate of metabolism of the drugs [59].

6.7 Toxicity of Vitamin B_6

Animal studies have shown that vitamin B_6 is potentially neurotoxic, causing peripheral neuropathy, with ataxia, muscle weakness and loss of balance in dogs given 200 mg pyridoxine/kg body weight for 40–75 days, and the development of a swaying gait and ataxia within 9 days at a dose of 300 mg/kg body weight [60, 61]. At the lower dose of 50 mg/kg body weight there are no clinical signs of toxicity, but histologically there is loss of myelin in dorsal nerve roots. At higher doses there is widespread neuronal damage, with loss of myelin and degeneration of sensory fibres in peripheral nerves, the dorsal columns of the spinal cord and the descending tract of the trigeminal nerve. The clinical signs of toxicity after 200–300 mg vitamin B_6/kg body weight regress within three months after the withdrawal of these massive doses, but sensory nerve conduction velocity, which decreases during the development of the neuropathy, does not recover fully [62].

In 1983, sensory neuropathy was reported [63] in seven patients who had been taking between 2–7000 mg of pyridoxine/day for several months for a variety of reasons. On withdrawal of the vitamin supplements there was considerable recovery of neuronal function, although there was some residual nerve damage in some patients. In a later study, giving 1 or 3 g vitamin B_6/day to healthy volunteers, electrophysiological and clinical abnormalities developed at the same time, and developed sooner in subjects receiving the higher dose of the vitamin. Symptoms continued to progress for 2–3 weeks after cessation of the supplements before regressing, although plasma concentrations of pyridoxal phosphate had returned to normal.

There has been one report of the development, within 2 years, of sensory neuropathy in an infant with vitamin B_6 dependent seizures treated with 2000 mg/day, but over the following 16 years the neuropathy did not progress [64]. However, most reports of patients with vitamin B_6 dependency diseases do not mention sensory neuropathy. One study has reported electrophysiological and neurological examination of 17 homocystinuric patients who had been treated with 200–500 mg vitamin B_6/day for 10–24 years; there was no evidence of neuropathy [65].

None of the studies in which there has been objective neurological examination has shown any evidence of sensory nerve damage at intakes of vitamin B_6 below 200 mg/day, and most have shown adverse effects only at considerably higher levels of intake.

One study [66] has suggested that relatively modest doses of vitamin B_6 may cause sensory nerve damage. Women who were taking 50–100 mg vitamin B_6/day for premenstrual syndrome were specifically asked to report symptoms such as tingling in the fingers, which might be interpreted as evidence of sensory neuropathy; a significant number of those taking 50 mg/day reported such symptoms. However, there was no neurological examination of any of the subjects, and no patients with similar premenstrual symptoms but not taking vitamin B_6 were asked the same questions. By contrast, a retrospective examination of the records of 630 women who had received 40–200 mg of vitamin B_6 for treatment of premenstrual syndrome found no reports of symptoms that suggested peripheral neuropathy.

The mechanism of nerve damage caused by vitamin B_6 supplements is not known. It is unlikely that pyridoxal phosphate itself is responsible. In patients with hypophosphatasia (lack of plasma alkaline phosphatase plasma concentrations of pyridoxal phosphate are very considerably higher than normal, even at normal intakes of the vitamin. However, the On-line Mendelian Inheritance in Man database [67] lists seizures as the only neurological sign in the (autosomal recessive) infant and childhood forms of the disease, and no neurological signs at all in the (autosomal dominant) adult form of the disease. Furthermore, plasma concentrations of pyridoxal phosphate do not rise above about 1000 nmol/l (10–15-fold higher than normal) even at very high levels of intake of the vitamin. However, plasma concentrations of pyridoxal and 4-pyridoxic acid do continue to increase with increasing intakes of the vitamin. This suggests that pyridoxal (or perhaps 4-pyridoxic acid) rather than pyridoxal phosphate, may be neurotoxic. Studies with cells in culture also support a cytotoxic effect of pyridoxal.

While there is no doubt that vitamin B_6 is neurotoxic in gross excess, there is considerable controversy over the way in which toxicological data have been translated into limits on the amounts that may be sold freely as 'nutritional supplements'. This appears to have been achieved by the application of standard toxicology safety margins, and taking as the upper safe limit of intake one percent of the 'no adverse effect level'. While this is appropriate for setting limits on additives and contaminants, it can be argued that it is not appropriate as a basis for setting limits on a nutrient; indeed for many nutrients an upper limit of intake established in this way would be below the average requirement to prevent deficiency. There is little evidence, apart from the report of an uncontrolled study, that intakes of up 200–500 mg vitamin B_6/day for prolonged periods, are associated with any adverse effects); clinical signs of neuropathy are associated with higher levels of intake, typically in excess of 1000 mg/day.

There is little convincing evidence that supplements of vitamin B_6 above levels to prevent deficiency have any beneficial effects, although a considerable number of women report or believe that supplements relieve the symptoms of the premenstrual syndrome. Equally, there is little convincing evidence that the levels of intake that are suggested or believed to be beneficial in treating the premenstrual syndrome are associated with any significant toxic hazard.

6.8 References

1. Department of Health. Committee on Toxicity of Chemicals In Food, Consumer Products and the Environment. Statement on vitamin B_6 (pyridoxine) toxicity. http://www.open.gov.uk/doh/hef/B_6.htm. 1997
2. Ink SL, Henderson LM. Vitamin B_6 metabolism. *Annual Review of Nutrition* 1984; 4: 455–470
3. Bender DA. Oestrogens and vitamin B_6 – actions and interactions. *World Review of Nutrition and Dietetics* 1987; 51: 140–88

4. Allgood VE, Cidlowski JA. Vitamin B_6 modulates transcriptional activation by multiple members of the steroid hormone receptor superfamily. *Journal of Biological Chemistry* 1992; 267: 3819–3824
5. Wiss O, Weber F. Biochemical pathology of vitamin B_6 deficiency. *Vitamins and Hormones* 1964; 22: 495–501
6. Department of Health. Report on Health and Social Subjects no 41: Dietary Reference Values for Food Energy and Nutrients for the United Kingdom. 1991, London, HMSO
7. National Research Council. Recommended Dietary Allowances 10th Edition. 1989, Washington, National Academy Press
8. Bender DA. Vitamin B_6 requirements and recommendations. *European Journal of Clinical Nutrition* 1989; 43: 289–300
9. Verhoef P, Stampfer MJ. Prospective studies of homocysteine and cardiovascular disease. *Nutrition Reviews* 1995; 3: 283–288
10. Selhub J, Jacques PF, Wilson PW, Rush D, Rosenberg IH. Vitamin status and intake as primary determinants of homocysteinemia in an elderly population. *Journal of the American Medical Association* 1993; 270: 2693–2698
11. Rimm EB, Willett WC, Hu FB, Sampson L, Colditz GA, Manson JE, Hennekens C, Stampfer MJ. Folate and vitamin B_6 from diet and supplements in relation to risk of coronary heart disease among women. *Journal of the American Medical Association* 1998; 279: 359–364
12. Dierkes J, Kroesen M, Pietrzik K. Folic acid and vitamin B_6 supplementation in healthy young women. *International Journal of Vitamin and Nutrition Research* 1998; 68: 98–103
13. Ubbinck JB, Vermaak WJH, van der Merwe A, Becker PJ, Delport R, Potgieter HC. Vitamin requirements for the treatment of hyperhomocystinaemia in humans. *Journal of Nutrition* 1994; 124: 1927–1933
14. Ubbinck JB. The role of vitamins in the pathogenesis and treatment of hyperhomocyst(e)inaemia. *Journal of Inherited Metabolic Diseases* 1997; 20: 316–325
15. Homocysteine lowering trialists' collaboration. Lowering blood homocysteine with folic acid based supplements: meta-analysis of randomised trials. *British Medical Journal* 1998; 316: 894–898
16. Merrill AH, Henderson LM. Diseases associated with defects in vitamin B_6 metabolism or utilisation. *Annual Review of Nutrition* 1987; 7: 137–156
17. Bender DA. Non-nutritional uses of vitamin B_6. *British Journal of Nutrition* 1999; 81: 7–20
18. Rose DP. The influence of oestrogens on tryptophan metabolism in man. *Clinical Science* 1966; 31: 265–272
19. Meister A. On the transamination of enzymes. *Annals of the New York Academy of Sciences* 1990; 585: 13–31
20. Bender DA, Wynick D. Inhibition of kynureninase (L-kynurenine hydrolase, EC 3.7.1.3) by oestrone sulphate, an alternative explanation for abnormal results of tryptophan load tests in women receiving oestrogenic steroids. *British Journal of Nutrition* 1981; 45: 269–275
21. Wynn V, Doar JW. Some effects of oral contraceptives on carbohydrate metabolism. *Lancet* 1966; (ii) 715–719
22. Rose DP, Leklem JE, Brown RR, Linkswiler HM. Effect of oral contraceptives and vitamin B_6 deficiency on carbohydrate metabolism. *American Journal of Clinical Nutrition* 1975; 28: 872–878
23. Bender DA, Totoe L. Inhibition of tryptophan metabolism by oestrogens in the rat, a factor in the aetiology of pellagra. *British Journal of Nutrition* 1984; 51: 219–224
24. Kotake Y, Ueda T, Mori T, Igaki S, Hattori M. Abnormal tryptophan metabolism and experimental diabetes by xanthurenic acid. *Acta Vitaminologica et Enzymologica* 1975; 29: 236–239
25. Adams PW, Wynn V, Folkard J, Seed M. Influence of oral contraceptives, pyridoxine (vitamin B_6), and tryptophan on carbohydrate metabolism. *Lancet* 1976; (i) 759–764
26. Rao RH. Glucose tolerance in subclinical pyridoxine deficiency in man. *American Journal of Clinical Nutrition* 1983; 38: 440–444

27. Toyota T, Kai Y, Kakizaki M, Ohtsuka H, Shibata Y, Goto Y. The endocrine pancreas in pyridoxine deficient rats. *Tohoku Journal of Experimental Medicine* 1981; 134: 331–336
28. Rao KS, Mohan PS. Plasma somatomedin activity, growth hormone and insulin levels in vitamin B_6 deficient rats. *Hormone and Metabolic Research* 1982; 14: 580–582
29. Hayakawa M, Shibata M. The in vitro and in vivo inhibition of protein glycosylation and diabetic vascular basement membrane thickening by pyridoxal 5′-phosphate. *Journal of Nutritional Science and Vitaminology (Tokyo)* 1991; 37: 149–159
30. Solomon LR, Cohen K. Erythrocyte O_2 transport and metabolism and effects of vitamin B_6 therapy in type II diabetes mellitus. *Diabetes* 1989; 38: 881–886
31. Eiduson S, Yuwiler A, Eberle ED. The effect of pyridoxine deficiency on L-aromatic amino acid decarboxylase and tyrosine aminotransferase in developing rat brain. *Advances in Biochemical Psychopharmacology* 1972; 4:63–80
32. Perry TL, Yong VW, Kish SJ, Ito M, Foulks JG, Godolphin WJ, Sweeney VP. Neurochemical abnormalities in brains of renal failure patients treated by repeated hemodialysis. *Journal of Neurochemistry* 1985; 45: 1043–1048
33. Bender DA, Totoe L. High doses of vitamin B_6 are associated with inhibition of hepatic tryptophan metabolism and increased uptake of tryptophan into the brain. *Journal of Neurochemistry* 1984; 43: 733–736
34. Ritchie CD, Singkamani R. Plasma pyridoxal 5′-phosphate in women with the premenstrual syndrome. *Human Nutrition: Clinical Nutrition* 1986; 40: 75–80
35. van den Berg H, Louwerse ES, Bruinse HW, Thissen JT, Schrijver J. Vitamin B_6 status of women suffering from premenstrual syndrome. *Human Nutrition: Clinical Nutrition* 1986; 40: 441–450
36. Mira M, Stewart PM, Abraham SF. Vitamin and trace element status in premenstrual syndrome. *American Journal of Clinical Nutrition* 1988; 47: 636–641
37. Kleijnen J, Ter-Riet G, Knipschild P. Vitamin B_6 in the treatment of the premenstrual syndrome – a review. *British Journal of Obstetrics and Gynaecology* 1990; 97: 847–852
38. Hagen I, Nesheim BI, Tuntland T. No effect of vitamin B-6 against premenstrual tension. A controlled clinical study. *Acta Obstetrica et Gynecologica Scandinavica* 1985; 64: 667–670
39. Brent RL. Bendectin: review of the medical literature of a comprehensively studied human nonteratogen and the most prevalent tortogen litigen. *Reproductive Toxicology* 1995; 9: 337–349
40. Sahakian V, Rouse D, Sipes S, Rose N, Niebyl J. Vitamin B_6 is effective therapy for nausea and vomiting of pregnancy:, a randomized, double-blind placebo controlled study. *Obstetrics and Gynecology* 1991; 78: 33–36
41. Vutyavanich T, Wongtra-ngan S, Ruangsri R. Pyridoxine for nausea and vomiting of pregnancy, a randomized, double-blind, placebo controlled trial. *American Journal of Obstetrics and Gynecology* 1995; 173: 881–884
42. Ellis JM, Kishi T, Azuma J, Folkers K. Vitamin B_6 deficiency in patients with a clinical syndrome including the carpal tunnel defect. Biochemical and clinical response to therapy with pyridoxine. *Research Communications in Chemical Pathology and Pharmacology* 1976; 13: 743–757
43. Ellis JM, Folkers K. Clinical aspects of treatment of carpal tunnel syndrome with vitamin B_6. *Annals of the New York Academy of Sciences* 1990; 585: 302–320
44. Amadio PC. Carpal tunnel syndrome, pyridoxine, and the work place. *Journal of the Hand Surgeons of America* 1978; 12: 875–880
45. Stransky M, Rubin A, Lava NS, Lazaro RP. Treatment of carpal tunnel syndrome with vitamin B_6: a double blind study. *Southern Medical Journal* 1989; 82: 841–842
46. Dakshinamurti K, Lal KJ. Vitamins and hypertension. *World Review of Nutrition and Dietetics* 1992; 69: 40–73
47. Dakshinamurti K, LeBlanq WD, Herchl R, Havelicek V. Non-parallel changes in brain monoamines of pyridoxal deficient growing rats. *Experimental Brain Research* 1976; 26: 355–366
48. Paulose CS, Dakshinamurti K, Packer S, Stephens NL. Sympathetic stimulation and hypertension in the pyridoxine deficient adult rat. *Hypertension* 1998;11: 387–391

49. Lal KJ, Dakshinamurti K. The relationship between low calcium induced increase in systolic blood pressure and vitamin B_6. *Journal of Hypertension* 1995; 13: 327–332
50. Fregly MJ, Cade JR. Effect of pyridoxine and tryptophan, alone and combined, on the development of deoxycorticosterone acetate induced hypertension in rats. *Pharmacology* 1995; 50: 298–306
51. Lal KJ, Dakshinamurti K, Thliveris J. The effect of vitamin B_6 on the systolic blood pressure of rats in various animal models of hypertension. *Journal of Hypertension* 1996; 14: 355–363
52. Aybak M, Sermet A, Ayyildiz MO, Karakilcik AZ. Effect of oral pyridoxine hydrochloride supplementation on arterial blood pressure in patients with essential hypertension. *Arzneimittelforschung* 1995; 45: 1271–1273
53. Vilter RW. The vitamin B_6-hydrazide relationship. *Vitamins and Hormones* 1964; 22: 797–805
54. Snider DE. Pyridoxine supplementation during isoniazid therapy. *Tubercle* 1980; 61: 191–196
55. Bender DA, Russell Jones R. Isoniazid-induced pellagra despite vitamin-B_6 supplementation. *Lancet* 1979; (ii), 1125–1126
56. Bender DA, Earl CJ, Lees AJ. Niacin depletion in Parkinsonian patients treated with L-dopa, benserazide and carbidopa. *Clinical Science* 1979; 56: 89–93
57. Fellman JH, Roth ES. Inhibition of tyrosine aminotransferase activity by L-dihydroxyphenylalanine. *Biochemistry* 1971; 10: 408–414
58. Glenn GM, Krober MS, Kelly P, McCarty J, Weir M. Pyridoxine as therapy in theophylline induced seizures. *Veterinary and Human Toxicology* 1995; 37: 342–345
59. Hansson O, Sillanppaa M. Pyridoxine and serum concentration of phenytoin and phenobarbitone. *Lancet* 1976; (i) 256
60. Phillips WE, Mills JH, Charbonneau SM, Tryphonas L, Hatina GV, Zawidzka Z, Bryce FR, Munro IC. Subacute toxicity of pyridoxine hydrochloride in the beagle dog. *Toxicology and Applied Pharmacology* 1978; 44: 323–333
61. Krinke G, Schaumburg HH, Spencer PS, Suter J, Thomann O, Hess R. Pyridoxine megavitaminosis produces degeneration of peripheral sensory neurons (sensory neuronopathy) in the dog. *Neurotoxicology* 1980; 2: 13–24
62. Schaeppi U, Krinke G. Pyridoxine neuropathy: correlation of functional tests and neuropathology in beagle dogs treated with large doses of vitamin B_6. *Agents and Actions* 1982; 12: 575–582
63. Schaumburg H, Kaplan J, Windebank A, Vick N, Rasmus S, Pleasure D, Brown MJ. Sensory neuropathy from pyridoxine abuse. A new megavitamin syndrome. *New England Journal of Medicine* 1983; 309: 445–448
64. McLachlan RS, Brown WF. Pyridoxine dependent epilepsy with iatrogenic sensory neuronopathy. *Canadian Journal of Neurological Science* 1995; 22: 50–51
65. Mpofu C, Alani SM, Whitehouse C, Fowler B, Wraith JE. No sensory neuropathy during pyridoxine treatment in homocystinuria. *Archives of Disease in Childhood* 1991; 66: 1081–1082
66. Dalton K, Dalton MJ. Characteristics of pyridoxine overdose neuropathy syndrome. *Acta Neurologica Scandinavica* 1987; 76: 8–11
67. On-Line Mendelian Inheritance in Man http://www3.ncbi.nlm.nih.gov/Omim/

7 Folic Acid and Disease Prevention: A Long Day's Journey Into Light

Christopher Schorah

7.1 Introduction

For many years it was believed that our diets need only provide enough of a particular vitamin to prevent the occurrence of severe deficiency disease. As most people in developed societies ate considerably more than this, there was complacency about our vitamin intake. Suggestions that requirements should be greater than those preventing overt deficiency, were often treated with disdain and contempt by the nutritional establishment. It was this attitude that fuelled the scientific shindy which greeted the publication of research indicating that intakes of folic acid [1] considerably higher than those preventing overt deficiency would prevent some serious birth defects [2]. In all, a long trek was needed to establish that this was indeed the case [3]. This is the story of that journey. Recent evidence indicating that increased intakes of folate may bring even more health benefits than the prevention of congenital malformations is also considered.

7.2 Folate Prevention of Neural Tube Defects

In the winter of 1944/45, the Dutch were having a hard time of it. In support of the allied landings in Normandy, there had been a strike in Holland and this, and the response of the occupying forces to the strike, had prevented distribution of food. By the time the issue was resolved, Holland was in the grip of a particularly hard winter, the canals had frozen and food distribution was very difficult. This resulted in what has become known as the Dutch Hunger Winter [4]. It was a short, sharp famine, lasting at its severest, about 3 months. Because social, scientific and medical facilities remained largely intact, aspects of the effect of the famine on health have been recorded. This is particularly true with regard to pregnancy [4].

---

[1] The metabolism of folic acid is complex and there are many different naturally occurring metabolites [1] most of which, unlike folic acid itself, occur in food. These are referred to collectively as folate. Folic acid, or pteroylmonoglutamate, is the specific form of folate used by the pharmaceutical industry in supplements, and the food industry for food fortification, and when that term is used here, it will denote that form of folate only.

The findings contained within these records were perhaps surprising in that short, severe food deprivation seemed to have relatively little effect on the outcome of pregnancy. Birth rate was considerably reduced, probably due to amenorrhoea, and many children were small-for-dates. However, these infants grew rapidly when the food supply improved, and seem to have suffered no long term ill effects from their deprivation. The only indication of permanent disadvantage was evidence which showed a significant increase in the prevalence of some malformations of the central nervous system, known as neural tube defects (NTD). These malformations occur very early in pregnancy, probably between the 20th and 28th day following conception, and are caused by a failure of the developing neural tube to close properly. If the lesion is towards the posterior end of the tube, which will eventually form the spine, then the condition is known as spina-bifida; if anterially, where the brain will develop, then the malformation is anencephaly, which is an absence of the fore-brain. Anencephalics do not survive, but children with spina bifida can live well into their teens and beyond. However, this malformation often results in major disability, with paralysis below the site of the lesion, double incontinence, and hydrocephalus, due to impaired flow of spinal fluids. The findings in Holland were not the first to suggest an association of the condition with poor nutrition. In the United Kingdom, social class and geographic differences in the prevalence of NTD, suggested a link with socio-economic disadvantage [5]. This association with poverty does not necessarily imply poor nutrition as the cause, because a number of environmental factors, such as infection [6], soft water [7], and the consumption of blighted potatoes [8], can also be associated with disadvantage. However, the findings in Holland firmly implicated a nutritional component, particularly as the malformation was most common when the height of the famine coincided with early pregnancy. There was also an indication that the nutritional deficiency could focus on folic acid, because there was evidence of disturbed maternal folate metabolism at the end of pregnancies associated with NTD [9].

Together, these associations began to make an increasingly powerful case for undernutrition as a causal factor in NTD, and to clarify the situation, Smithells and colleagues [10] undertook a detailed investigation of the nutrition of mothers in early pregnancy, close to the time of neural tube closure. Well over 1,000 women were investigated for approximately 20 nutritional indices. The only differences found in those who subsequently had an NTD -affected infant, were lower maternal levels of red cell folic acid, and white cell vitamin C.

It is biological plausible to implicate deficiencies of folic acid in the cause of NTD. The vitamin is required for the synthesis of bases found in DNA and is therefore crucial to cell division (Fig. 1). Early in pregnancy, at the time of closure of the neural tube, the cells in the neural folds are dividing very rapidly, and hence they need a good supply of components required for the synthesis of nucleic acids. It is also a very critical time in the supply of nutrients to the foetus. At the start of neural tube closure the fetal heart is not yet beating, and nutrients need to diffuse from a digest of maternal cells, through maternal and embryonic tissue to the site of their activity. The growth of the developing foetus is beginning to compromise this nutrient supply by increasing the diffusion path

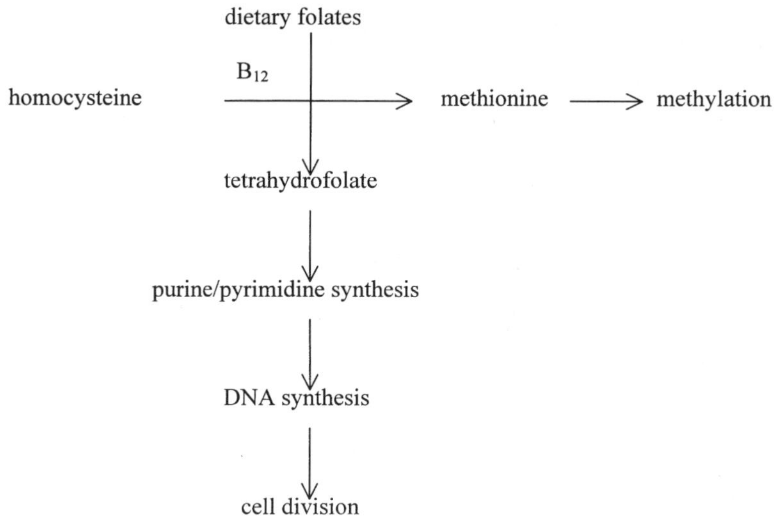

Fig. 1. Simplified scheme outlining the metabolic roles of folate

beyond efficient limits, but the development of an effective circulation of fetal blood is still some days away [11].

If impaired folate supply was indeed a cause of NTD, then increased intakes of the vitamin could be preventive. Our research group, therefore, undertook a series of periconceptional multi-vitamin intervention studies with the supplement Pregnavite forte F (Bencard) [2,12–15], which provided approximately the recommended daily intake for pregnancy of most vitamins, including folic acid, but not vitamin B_{12}. This was, therefore, not a high dose regimen, but one which could be considered physiological. The studies were undertaken in women who had already had at least one infant with NTD and who where, therefore, at increased risk of a recurrence (about 5% risk). The results were striking. There was an 80% reduction in the prevalence of the condition in women who received the supplements, whilst the rate in the unsupplemented group was about that which would be expected for a high-risk population. However, because the study was not randomised, it was suggested that the findings could be due to the selection process which had inadvertently led to a group of women at low risk of recurrence being chosen for supplementation [16–19]. Quite rightly, randomised intervention studies with vitamins were planned, but before the findings of these studies were known, further publications and more detailed analysis of the data from the Smithells group, indicated that selection bias was a very unlikely explanation for the findings [5,20]. This was particularly so in Northern Ireland, where periconceptional multi-vitamin supplementation, extending with time to an increasing proportion of women at high risk for NTD, had almost eliminated recurrence of the condition in the province.

The controversy was finally laid to rest when the Medical Research Council published the findings of their randomised intervention study which, with its four arms including folic acid alone and multivitamins without folate, was clearly able to show that folic acid, and not other vitamins, dramatically decreased the *recurrence* of NTD [3]. The results of a large randomised intervention study in Hungary, followed almost immediately afterwards and showed that multivitamin intervention was also able to reduce the *occurrence* of NTD in the general population [21].

It is now clear that appropriate folate supplementation will prevent a large proportion of these malformations. Because the malformation occurs very early in pregnancy, supplementation needs to start before conception. Supplementation starting after confirmation of pregnancy will be beyond the critical time point when the neural tube closes, and will almost certainly by ineffective [22].

Following these findings important public health issues arose for example, how much folate is needed in the diet to maximise the prevention of NTD? How can health professionals ensure that women of child bearing age receive this in their diet before they conceive? Before addressing these questions, other situations where increased folate intake has been implicated in the prevention of disease must be considered.

7.3 Other Congenital Malformations and Folate

If the action of folate is indeed one of encouraging fetal cell division and provision of adequate cell material for the closure of the neural tube, it could have an effect on other malformations? Czeizel's study [21] of prevention of NTD *occurrence* was sufficiently large to look at its impact on all malformations. The results indicated that not only was there a significant effect on the prevalence NTD, but all types of malformation were reduced by about 50% [23]. These findings require confirmation, as a multivitamin preparation was used, but this may now not be possible because withholding folate in an intervention study in pregnancy is no longer ethically acceptable because of its ability to prevent NTD.

7.4 Folate, Homocysteine and Occlusive Vascular Disease

For many years it has been known that patients who are homozygous for homocystinuria, are at increased risk of occlusive vascular disease (OVD). These patients have extremely high levels of plasma homocysteine, due to defects in the metabolism of this amino acid. More recently it has been shown that even moderate elevations of plasma homocysteine are associated with the condition. Reviews of a large number of retrospective epidemiological surveys and a few prospective studies, now indicate that homocysteine is an independent risk factor for stroke, ischaemic heart disease and peripheral vascular disease [24, 27]. It is not known whether the elevated homocysteine is causal, or just associated with the condition. However, recent evidence from prospective studies showing that the highest homocysteine levels are associated with both the most severe disease and the most rapid rate of disease progression, indicates that homocysteine is a causative agent [28–31]. If this is the case, then it could account for about 30% of risk of OVD.

Homocysteine is metabolised partially by conversion to methionine (Fig. 1) and this step requires methylation by folate. It is not, therefore, surprising that the body's supply of folate is inversely related to plasma levels of homocysteine [26, 32–37]. This is true whether considering the circulating levels of folate or folate intake. Further, several recent studies have shown that physiological and supraphysiological increases in folate intake are able to reduce plasma homocysteine levels [38–41] illustrating that there is a simple and non-toxic way of decreasing a potentially atherogenic agent. If this potential is realised, then an increased supply of folate, not only to a relatively small group of women who are about to conceive, but to the general population, will significantly impact the prevalence of a major disease. Again, as with folate prevention of NTD, the central issue will be, how much folate is needed, and how is it to be provided?

7.5 Folate Requirements and Provision

Table 1 gives an approximate estimation of the prevalence of NTD at different intakes of folate. It is clear from this that folate intakes less than 200 μg should be avoided in all pregnancies, and that an average intake, which is feasible and which will move towards maximising prevention, is about 500 μg per day. As discussed earlier, recent publications suggest that such an increase in intake could also have a significant impact on OVD, through its effect on plasma homocysteine [38–41]. When one realises that inadequate folate supply has also been associated with an increased risk of some cancers [45], although not strongly, and is definitely associated with a reduced prevalence of all malformations [23], it would seem that an intake of 500 μg of folate each day for everyone is the ideal which should be an achievable goal. First of all, this means that individuals who are at particularly high risk of either fetal malformation, because of previous abnormal births, or occlusive vascular disease, because of particular high homocysteine levels, should receive appropriate folate supplements. But these are specific cases. They will be identified from their medical history, and can receive individual therapy accordingly. What about those who have no history of fetal malformation or occlusive vascular disease? There are potentially three ways adequate folate supply can be achieved in the general population. These are: changed diet, supplements and food fortification.

Table 1. Estimated first trimester prevalence of NTD in the UK at different intakes and tissue reserves of folate. Derived from data in references [2, 10, 21, 42–44]

Erythrocyte folate (μg/l)	Folate intake (μg/d)	Estimated NTD revalence/1000 pregnancies
<150	<200	8.0
150–400	200–400	1.5
>400	400–600	<0.5

7.6 Changed Diet

Table 2 gives an outline of food sources of folate. Whilst small amounts of folate are present in many foods, rich sources tend to be in foods that are not commonly eaten. A diet that contained this author's recommended average of 500 μg per day, would need to be high in liver or liver products, pulses and dark green vegetables. This is neither a typical diet, nor one that is likely to be popular. There is also evidence that food-forms of folate are less biologically available than pteroylmonoglutamate, the form of folate used in supplements and food fortification. It is thus almost impossible for dietary modifications alone to achieve an adequate folate supply at the present time. Health professionals do need to continue to recommend increased consumption of fruit and vegetables, because this diet is associated with reduced risk of cancer [46] and possibly ischaemic heart disease, but this is not going to maximise disease prevention through increased folate supply.

7.7 Supplements

Supplements of folic acid are very effective as indicated by their ability to prevent NTD in the multivitamin intervention studies [2, 3, 12–15, 21]. They are cheap and, at the level suggested, non-toxic. They will, however, only be taken by those who are both aware and understand the need. The syndrome of socioeconomic disadvantage dictates that, those who most need an increased supply because of poor diet are least likely to take supplements. A further example of ineffectiveness of supplements are unplanned pregnancies, said to be about 40% of all pregnancies in the UK [47, 48]. A woman is very unlikely to take a supplement for pregnancy when she is not intending to conceive. The poor penetration of supplement use has been reported. Figures show that two years after the publication of the MRC study, supplement use was very low in women of childbearing age, and had still only risen to about 30% of this population, even after a major government education initiative [48].

Table 2. Examples of foods containing relatively high levels of folate

Folate sources
Dark green vegetables: broccoli, spinach, Brussel sprouts, asparagus, spring greens
Pulses: lentils, mung beans, red kidney beans, chick peas
Offal: liver, pâté, kidney
Concentrated sources: Bovril, Marmite, yeast

7.8 Food Fortification

Food fortification is the only alternative that is likely to produce a real impact on folate intake and disease prevention. Table 3 gives a summary of how the fortification of staple foods such as cereals and bread could achieve my suggested minimum intake of folic acid in almost the whole population, and an increase in average intakes to 500 μg per day. The only argument against such a policy is that a significant number of individuals who would receive an increased folate supply would not need it. This argument only has weight if this is detrimental. There is no evidence that an increased intake of folic acid of up to 1 mg per day, and particularly if taken in divided doses through food fortification, would have any detrimental impact on the population. The diversionary arguments or "red herrings" that have been used to distract the UK Government's decision making bodies from going ahead with food fortification, include the potential for folic acid to increase convulsions, and mask vitamin B_{12}. deficiency. Folate intakes that would have any tendency to produce these effects are above 1 mg, taken as a single pharmacological dose, indeed the threshold is probably closer to 5 mg than 1 mg [51]. It is estimated that through voluntary supplement use during the last 20 years, an increasing proportion of the population of the USA has been consuming folate at a higher intake than 500 μmg per day however no increased prevalence of epilepsy or masked vitamin B_{12} deficiency has been recorded in this group.

Table 3. Proposals for maximising folate prevention of disease by food fortification

Suggested new daily folate requirements		
All intakes	>200 μg/d	
Average intake	500 μg/d	
Proposed mandatory folic acid fortification of food to achieve requirements		
Cereals	150 μg/portion	
Bread	70 μg/slice	
Chapati flour	70 μg/chapati	
Effects of fortification on daily folate intakes (μg/d)		
Minimum (2.5th percentile of population)		
Current[a] (without proposed fortification)		125
Cereals (increase with proposed fortification)		25
Bread[b] (increase with proposed fortification)		50
Total (with fortification)		200
Average (50th percentile of population)		
Current[a] (without proposed fortification)		255
Cereals[c] (increase with proposed fortification)		70
Bread[b] (increase with proposed fortification)		175
Total (with fortification)		500

[a] See [49, 50].
[b] Women of child bearing age consume 2.5 slices/day and 99% eat bread (50).
[c] 70% of population eat cereals, current average level of fortification is 50 μg/serving.

Finally, overt folate-deficiency anaemia (megablastosis) is not uncommon in the sick elderly [52]. Food fortification could effectively eliminate this problem.

7.9 Conclusions

Increased folate intake in the diet at high physiological doses will considerably reduce the prevalence of NTD and probably have an impact on other major malformations. It could also prevent up to 30% of cases of OVD and would virtually eliminate folate deficiency anaemia. A good public health policy would recommend consumption of green vegetables demand mandatory fortification of food with folate and provide supplements for those at especially high risk.

The USA is already fortifying flour with folic acid, although the levels need to be increased. It is timely that the United Kingdom and the rest of Europe followed suit. Indeed, if homocysteine is found to be a causal risk factor for occlusive vascular disease, there will be no excuse for not immediately adopting a mandatory food-fortification policy in the UK and the rest of Europe.

7.10 References

1. Schorah CJ. Critical glossary: folic acid. In: Dobbing J (ed*) Prevention of Spina Bifida and other Neural Tube Defects.* London: Academic Press; pp 241–242, 1983
2. Smithells RW, Sheppard S, Schorah CJ, Seller MJ, Nevin NC, Harris R, Read AP, Fielding DW. Possible prevention of neural tube defects by periconceptional vitamin supplementation. *Lancet* 1980; i: 339–340
3. MRC Vitamin Study Research Group. Prevention of neural tube defects: results of the MRC vitamin study. *Lancet* 1991; 338: 131–137
4. Stein Z, Susser M, Gerhart S, Marolla F. Famine and Human Development: The Dutch Hunger Winter of 1944–1945. *London: Oxford University Press,* 1975
5. Schorah CJ, Smithells RW. A possible role for periconceptional multivitamin supplementation in the prevention of the recurrence of neural tube defects. In: Bendich A, Butterworth CE (eds) *Micronutrients in Health and the Prevention of Disease* New York: Marcel Dekker Inc, pp 263–285, 1991
6. Record RG. Anencephalus in Scotland. *Br J Preventitive and Social Medicine* 1961; 15: 93–105
7. Stocks P. Incidence of congenital malformations in the regions of England and Wales. *Br J Preventitive and Social Medicine* 1970; 24: 67–72
8. Renwick JH. Hypothesis: anencephaly and spina bifida are usually preventable by avoidance of a specific but unidentified substance present in certain potato tubers. *Br J Preventitive and Social Medicine* 1972; 26: 67–72
9. Hibbard ED, Smithells RW. Folic acid metabolism and human embryopathy. *Lancet* 1965; i: 1254
10. Smithells RW, Sheppard S, Schorah CJ. Vitamin deficiencies and neural tube defects. *Arch Disease in Childhood* 1976; 51: 944–950
11. Beck F. The use of whole embryo culture of the rat in experimental study of human birth defects. In: Dobbing J (ed) Prevention of Spina Bifida and other Neural Tube Defects. *London: Academic Press,* 23–40, 1983
12. Smithells RW, Sheppard S, Schorah CJ, Seller MJ, Nevin NC, Harris R, Read AP, Fielding DW. Apparent prevention of neural tube defects by periconceptional vitamin supplementation. *Arch Disease in Childhood* 1981; 56: 911–918

13. Smithells RW, Nevin NC, Seller MJ, Sheppard S, Harris R, Read AP, Fielding DW, Walker S, Schorah CJ, Wild J. Further experience of vitamin supplementation for prevention of neural tube defect recurrences. *Lancet* 1983; i: 1027–1031
14. Schorah CJ, Wild J, Hartley R, Sheppard S, Smithells RW. The effect of periconceptional supplementation on blood vitamin concentrations in women at recurrence risk for neural tube defect. *Br J Nutr* 1983; 49: 203–211
15. Smithells RW, Sheppard S, Wild J, Schorah CJ. Prevention of neural tube defects recurrences in Yorkshire: final report. *Lancet* 1989; ii: 498–499
16. Knox EG. Vitamin supplementation and neural tube defects. *Lancet* 1983; ii: 39
17. Oakley GP, Adms MJ, James LM. Vitamins and neural tube defects. *Lancet* 1983; ii: 798–799
18. Elwood JM. Can vitamins prevent neural tube defects? *Canadian Med Assoc J* 1983; 129: 1088–1092
19. Wald NJ, Polani PE. Neural tube defects and vitamins: the need for a randomised clinical trial. *Br J Obstet & Gynae* 1984; 91: 516–523
20. Wild J, Read AP, Sheppard S, Seller MJ, Smithells RW, Nevin NC, Schorah CJ, Fileding DW, Walker S, Harris R. Recurrent neural tube defects, risk factors and vitamins. *Arch Disease in Childhood* 1986; 61: 440–444
21. Czeizel AE, Dudas I. Prevention of the first occurrence of neural-tube defects by periconceptional vitamin supplementation. *New Engl J Med* 1992; 327: 1832–1836
22. Sheppard S, Nevin NC, Seller MJ, Wild J, Smithells RW, Reed AP, Harris R, Fielding DW, Schorah CJ. Neural tube defect recurrence after 'partial' vitamin supplementation. *J Med Gen* 1989; 26: 326–329
23. Czeizel AE. Prevention of congenital abnormalities by periconceptional multivitamin supplementation. *Br Med J* 1993; 306: 1645–1648
24. Malinow MR. Hyperhomocysteinaemia. A common and easily reversible risk factor for occlusive atherosclerosis. *Circulation* 1990; 81: 2004–2006
25. Ueland PM, Refsum H, Brattström L. Plasma homocysteine and cardiovascular disease. In: Francis BR (ed) *Atherosclerosis Cardiovascular Disease, Homeostasis and Endothelial Function,* NY: Marcel Dekker, pp 183–235, 1992
26. Boers GH. Hyperhomocysteinaemia: a newly recognised risk factor for vascular disease. *Neth J Med* 1994; 45: 34–41
27. Masser PA Taylor LM, Porter JM. Importance of elevated plasma homocysteine levels as a risk factor for atherosclerosis. *Ann Thorc Surg* 1994; 58: 1240–1246
28. Taylor L, DeFrang RD, Harris EJ, Portor JM. The association of elevated plasma homocysteine with progression of symptomatic peripheral arterial disease. *J Vas Surg* 1991; 13: 128–136
29. Stampter MJ, Malinow MR, Willett WC, Newcomer LM, Upson B, Ullmann D, Tishler DB, Hennekens CH. A prospective study of plasma homocysteine and risk of myocardial infarction in US physicians. *J Am Med Ass* 1992; 268: 877–881
30. Boushey CJ, Beresford SA, Omenn GS, Motulsky AG. A quantitative assessment of plasma homocysteine as a risk factor for vascular disease. Probable benefits of increasing folic acid intakes. *J Am Med Ass* 1995; 274: 1049–1057
31. Wald NJ, Watt HC. Law MR, Weir DG, McPartlin JM, Scott JM. Homocysteine and ischaemic heart disease: results of a prospective study with implications regarding prevention. *Arch Intern Med* 1998; 158: 862–867
32. Pancharuniti N, Lewis CA, Sauberlich HE, Perkins LL, Go RC, Alvarez JO, Macaluso M, Acton RT, Copeland RB, Cousins AL. Plasma homocysteine, folate and vitamin B_{12}. concentrations and risk for early onset coronary artery disease. *Am J Clin Nutr* 1994; 59: 940–948
33. Wilken DEL, Dudman NPB, Tyrrell PA, Robertson MR. Folic acid lowers elevated plasma homocysteine in chronic renal insufficiency: possible implications for prevention of vascular disease. *Metabolism* 1988; 37: 697–670
34. Arnadottir M, Brattström L, Simonsen O, Thysell H, Hultberg B, Anderson A, Nilsson-Ehle P. The effect of high dose, pyridoxide and folic acid suplementation on serum lipid and plasma homocysteine concentration in dialysis patients. *Clin Nephrol* 1993; 40: 236–240

35. Bergmark C, Mansoor MA, Swedonborg J, de Faire V, Svardal AM, Ueland PM. Hyperhomocysteinaemia in patients operated for lower extremity ischaemic below the age of 50: effect of smoking and extent of disease. *Eur J Vasc Surg* 1993; 7: 391–396
36. Selhub J, Jacques PF, Wilson PWF, Rush D, Rosenberg IH. Vitamin status and intake as primary determinants of homocysteinaemia in an elderly population. *J Am Med Ass* 1993; 270: 2693–2698
37. Verhoef P, Stampfer MJ, Buring JE, Gaziano JM, Allen RH, Stabler SP, Reynolds RD, Kok FJ, Hennekens CH, Willett WC. Homocysteine metabolism and risk of myocardial infarction: relation with vitamins B B_{12} and folate. *Am J Epidemiol* 1996; 143: 845–859
38. Ubbink JB, Vermaak WJ, van der Merwe A, Becker PJ, Delport R, Potgieter HC. Vitamin requirements for the treatment of hyperhomocysteinemia. *J Nutr* 1994; 124: 1927–1933
39. Guttormsen AB, Ueland PM, Nasthus J, Nygard O, Schneede J, Vollset SE, Refsum H. Determinants and vitamin responsiveness of intermediate hyperhomocysteinemia (> of = 40 μmol/l). The Hordaland Homocysteine Study. *J Clin Invest* 1996; 98: 2174–2183
40. Ward M, McNulty H, McPartlin JM, Strain JJ, Weir D, Scott JM. The response of plasma homocysteine to low-dose pteroylglutamic (folic) acid supplementation in healthy male subjects. *Proc Nutr Soc* 1997; 56: 148 A
41. Schorah CJ, Devitt H, Lucock M, Dowell AC. The responsiveness of plasma homocysteine to small increases in dietary folic acid: a primary care study. *Euro J Clin Nutr* 1998; 52: 407–411
42. Rogozinski H, Ankers C, Lennon D, Wild J, Schorah C, Sheppard S, Smithells RW. Folate nutrition in early pregnancy. *Human Nutrition: Applied Nutrition* 1983; 37 A: 357–364
43. Kirke PN, Molloy AM, Daly LE, Burke H, Weir DG, Scott JM. Maternal plasma folate and vitamin B_{12}. are independant risk factors for neural tube defects. *Quart J Clin Nutr* 1993; 86: 703–708
44. Daly LE, Kirke PN, Molloy A, Weir DG, Scott JM. Folate levels and neural tube defects: implications for prevention. *JAMA* 1995; 274: 1693–1702
45. Butterworth CE. Folate deficiency and cancer. In: Bendich A, Butterworth CE (eds) Micronutrients in health and Prevention of Disease. New York. Marcle Dekker, pp 165–183, 1991
46. Schorah CJ. Micronutrients, vitamins and cancer risk. *Vit Hormones* 1999; 57: 1–23
47. Becker GL. Folic acid and food fortification. *Food Processing* 1994; May: 41–44
48. Wild J, Sutcliffe M, Schorah CJ, Levene MI. Prevention of neural tube defects. *Lancet* 1997; 350: 30
49. Wild J. Seller MJ, Schorah CJ, Smithells RW. Investigation of folate intake and metabolism in women who had two pregnancies complicated by neural tube defects. *Br J Obstet Gynaecol* 1994; 101: 197–202
50. Wild J, Schorah CJ, Maude K, Levine MI. Folate intake in young women and their knowledge of pre-conceptional folate supplementation to prevent neural tube defects. Eur J Obstet Gynecol 1996; 70: 185–189
51. Dickinson CJ. Does folic acid harm people with B_{12} deficiency? *Quart J Med* 1995; 88: 357–364
52. Schorah CJ, Habibzadeh N. Folates in embryonic development and old age. In: Taylor TG, Jenkins NK (eds) *Proceedings XIII International Congress of Nutrition.* London: J Libbey, pp 457–460, 1986

8 The Addition of Micronutrients to Food

H. Frank Woods

8.1 Introduction

The practice of adding micronutrients to food with the objective of correcting a dietary deficiency, has its origins in the nineteenth century. In the twentieth century, mainly as a result of two World Wars, the practice has become widespread, extending beyond the aim of treating specific deciciency diseases to the objective of their prevention through the addition of micronutrients to certain dietary constituents. More recently attention has been given to the prevention of inherited and acquired disease through the use of micronutrient supplementation. There is, in addition, the emergence of the practice of adding micronutrients to foods as a marketing aid.

The purpose of this paper is to place the subject in its historical context and then to discuss the current state of affairs in the light of the nutritional aims of the practice, policy issues and the relevant legislation.

8.2 The Historical Background

Two concepts formulated during the nineteenth century are germain to the subject matter of this paper. One was the demonstration by Lunin that natural diets contain unknown factors, small amounts of which are necessary for life. The other was that Beri beri, which had been described in the seventeenth century, together with conditions such as rickets and scurvy, were deficiency diseases caused by the absence from the diet or a limited supply in the diet, of compounds which, at that time, were unidentified (the vitamins).

Thus, there emerged the principle that the human diet, in order to be optimal, must contain vitamins in addition to protein, fat, carbohydrate and minerals.

The effect of the application of the principles of scientific nutritional knowledge to the provision of an adequate diet can be discerned in the dietary policy adopted towards the end of the First World War. Initially, in Britain, following the creation of the Ministry of Food early in the War, little notice was taken of scientific advice on the constitution of the diet. However, after an attempt to introduce voluntary rationing of certain foodstuffs during the last eighteen months of the War rationing was introduced.

The contemporary scientific advice to Government had centred upon the total energy content of the diet and there was no emphasis upon its micronutrient content. However, some nutritional policies, although they were not formulated for that purpose, influenced the intake of vitamins and minerals. Thus, the introduction of "war bread" in 1916 made with flour of 76% extraction was followed by changes in the extraction rate which reached 92% in early 1918, falling later to 87%: the level at which it remained until controls ceased. The high extraction rate would have gone towards ensuring that iron consumption would have risen and the risk of Vitamin B_1 deficiency would have been lowered. There would have been an increased intake of nicotinic acid and riboflavin. On the other hand, in 1918, there was an inadequate supply of butter and margarine; the latter not being fortified with Vitamins A and D. The role of butter as a source of these vitamins had not yet been recognised. Thus, on the basis of these facts, it can be argued that any influence of policy upon the intake of micronutrients was largely fortuitous.

During the War, the diet had become poorer in calcium and more deficient in Vitamin D while its carbohydrate and, therefore, energy content had increased. Attempts were made to determine whether the eighteen month period of dietary restriction during rationing had resulted in a measurable nutritional effect upon the population as a whole or upon sub groups within it. An example was the estimation of the prevalence of rickets in children. Unfortunately there was no high quality information relating to the prevalence prior to 1917 which could provide a reference value. Anecdotal evidence that the incidence of rickets had risen was given by Corry Mann [1] and the work of Friend [2] established an adverse effect upon some aspects of the nutritional status of boys at Christs Hospital School although this group cannot be regarded as being representative of the population as a whole.

At the outbreak of the Second World War, the United Kingdom was properly prepared for the application of nutritional science to the feeding of its population. Plans for the rationing and distribution of food had been drawn up based upon the experience gained during the First World War. A guiding force in the policy was Sir Jack Drummond, who wrote two official papers which predicted the nutritional needs of the population in wartime with emphasis upon (economically) poorer subgroups contained within it. Drummond reviewed these documents in 1947 [3].

Professor Drummond's recommendations included advice regarding the fortification of margarine with Vitamins A and D; the addition of calcium carbonate to flour and the Vitamins Welfare Scheme which ensured an adequate intake of Vitamins A, C and D during pregnancy and early life.

The success of these policies established the value of the fortification of food and the use of food supplements and when, coupled to the rationing system, ensured that there was not only an equable distribution of food sufficient to supply the basic nutritional needs of the population but also a proper provision of vitamins and other micronutrients according to the then current state of nutritional knowledge.

The quantification of the success of the various measures is more problematical. There was no evidence of an increase in the increase of specific deficiency diseases during the Second World War and, in common with the findings during other major conflicts such as the First World War and the Franco-Prussian War, the "health" of the nation as gauged by a decreased prevalence of Diabetes Mellitus and Coronary Heart Disease was improved [4].

8.3 Some Definitions

The terminology applied to the process of adding micronutrients to food is complex. Definitions of terms have been published by Codex Alimentarious [5] and other definitions have been set out in a monograph published by the Institute of Food Science & Technology [6] and the SCOOP Task Group Report [7]. The definitions included in Table 1 are an amalgam of those appearing in these publications and they have been constructed with the aim and object of presenting an unambiguous meaning for each term.

In the scientific literature and in general, the terms are often used out of context and in an interchangeable manner. For example, *fortification* and *enrichment* have been taken to mean the addition of a nutrient solely with the purpose of preventing or correcting a demonstrated deficiency of one or more nutrients in the population as a whole or in a specific group within the population. Alternatively, *fortification* has been defined as the addition of nutrients to foods other than cereals, *enrichment* being defined as the addition of nutrients to cereals [8].

Table 1. The definitions of terms used to describe the process of adding micronutrients to food. These definitions are based upon those given in [5–7]

Term	Definition
Restoration	The addition to a food of nutrients lost during manufacture or processing in quantities which result in the full or partial presence in the food to that level in the edible portion of the food present before processing, storage or handling
Fortification	The addition of nutrients to foods irrespective of whether or not it is normally contained in the food for the purpose of preventing or correcting a demonstrated deficiency of one or more nutrients in the population or specific groups within the population
Enrichment	The addition of a nutrient (or nutrients) already present in the food in order to make it a richer source
Standardisation	The addition of nutrients in order to compensate for natural, e.g. seasonal, variations in nutrient content
Substitution	The addition of a nutrient to a substitute product to the level in the food which it is designed to resemble

8.4 The Rationale for the Addition of Nutrients to Food

It could be argued that, on the basis of a knowledge of the diet currently consumed in developed countries, sufficient nutrients would be supplied in that diet to support development, growth and the maintenance of health in adult life. This contention is indirectly strengthened by the wide availability and variety of foods available.

However, when the results of nutritional surveys are considered the data indicate that, within the population, there are sub groups who appear to have mineral and vitamin intakes below those recommended nationally. The data for the Member States of the European Community based upon nutritional surveys show that each has at least two micronutrients whose intakes are below those recommended so far as parts of their population are concerned [7]. Comparisons between Member States are fraught with difficulty because the population groups considered were very divergent as were the sizes of the studies, the methodology for assessing food consumption and the criteria used in the evaluations. It is of note that the surveys included the consumption of fortified foods with the implication that, for some nutrients, the fortifications carried out are not effective in correcting intakes which are less than those recommended. Additional difficulties when considering the data, are the differences in nationally applied nutritional standards and a gross lack of information concerning the nutritional status of population groups.

8.5 Policy Considerations

The proposition put forward in the previous section that a varied diet can provide the nutrients required for both development and the maintenance of normal health has to undergo modification so far as certain population subgroups are concerned, most probably because of changing eating habits, such as the increased consumption of snack and pre-prepared food coupled to less food preparation in the home. The lowered energy expenditure in the elderly may, as a secondary effect, result in an inadequate intake of micronutrients [9, 10].

Nutritional research has provided much information as to the Recommended Daily Allowance (RDA[1]) for mincronutrients and these can be used as a benchmark for fixing the extent of fortification as well as indicating the need for fortification where the diet is not providing the RDA. There may also be a mismatch between the nutritional status and the intake of a particular nutrient.

Currently attention is focused upon the causal relationships between the provision of individual nutrients and disease with special emphasis upon vitamins and minerals. One example is that of the relationship between the risk of the development of neural tube defects and the intake of folic acid by women of

[1] RDA – Recommended Daily Allowance. The amounts of the nutrient sufficient or more than sufficient for the nutritional needs of practically all healthy persons in a population.

child-bearing age [11, 12]. The scientific aspects of this subject are considered in the chapter written by Scorah. However, this example provides a good basis for the discussion of policy and practice.

If the given fact is that there is a benefit to be gained from increasing folic acid intake so far as the prevention of neural tube defects is concerned, the policy objective can be formulated as a question: *"How can the increased intake be achieved?"*

There are three practical routes which could be used in order to result in an increased intake of folic acid:

i) through nutrition education focused upon the target group within the population.
ii) via the fortification of food.
iii) the recommendation of the use of supplements.

For route (ii) there are alternative policies which are (a) compulsory addition of folic acid to certain foods; (b) a recommendation that folic acid is added to certain foods and (c) the permitting of the addition of folic acid to certain foods.

The choice as to which policy or policies to use must be informed by the science and once a policy has been adopted, it has to be modulated by safety and legislative considerations. The example of folic acid intake and neural tube defects also allows a discussion of the safety of fortification.

The excessive intake of micronutrients can be associated in a causal manner to adverse effects in man and these have been reviewed [13, 14]. In the case of folic acid there is the potential effect of masking the consequences of Vitamin B_{12} deficiency at high folic acid intakes, namely more than 1 mg/day. This could potentially have the effect of delaying the diagnosis of Vitamin B_{12} deficiency and make damage to the neurological system more likely to occur. This proposition has been contested in relation to the risk versus benefit assessment for folate administration in the context of the prevention of neural tube defects [15].

To complete the policy sequence further stages are necessary. The first is to determine whether fortification of foods with folate gives rise to increases in its intake and subsequently in the serum folate concentration. In the United States the fortification of cereals and grain with folic acid became mandatory in 1996; the Food and Drug Administration having laid down that cereal grain must be fortified to a level of 140 μm g per 100 grams of cereal grain [16]. The fortification process was to have been completed before 1st January 1998. Estimates suggested that women in the United States would, as a result, increase their intake of folic acid by 80 μg per day.

In order to determine whether serum folate levels had changed following food fortification, Lawrence et al. [17] analysed the results of serum folate determinations made in one clinical laboratory during a five year period (1994–1998 inclusive). Their analysis showed that the percentage of specimens with high folate values (> 20 μg/l) increased steadily from 1997, the year in which the percentage of specimens with low values (< 2.7 μg/l) began to decrease. There was an increase in the median folate concentration value during the period studied which also started in 1997. The authors concluded that serum folate levels are rising and that the fortification of food with folic acid was the most likely explanation for the increase. However, the results apply to a hospital population and, although the proportion of women in the population was 53%, the majority of those were not in the reproductive years and the analyses of the data did not include one by gender or by age.

In considering the general case estimates of the contribution made by the enrichment of foods with micronutrients to the dietary intake of vitamins and minerals are available. Thus, Lachance & Bauernfiend [18] demonstrated that enrichment contributed to the intake of some vitamins and iron in the United States of America. These authors also reviewed the position in countries where a shortage of micronutrients had resulted in the development of deficiency diseases and concluded that enrichment had improved the provision of micronutrients without there being concomitant data on the nutritional status of the populations of subgroups within them there are limited data showing the contribution of fortified foods to vitamin intake within the European Community. The figures for Vitamin A and Vitamin D are shown on Table 2. There is much variation between countries and it is clear that the supply of Vitamin A is much less dependent upon fortification than that of Vitamin D.

In theory, the consumption of staple foods, all of which were fortified, could lead to consumption of micronutrients in daily quantities which are several times the respective RDA for each compound. The risks associated with this are dependent upon the dose response effect relationship for each compound in relation to their toxic effects. However, there is little or no evidence of toxicity as a result of fortification alone.

8.6 Legislative Aspects of Micronutrients Addition to Food

The legislation governing the addition of micronutrients to food varies widely across the European Community. In the United Kingdom (where the definition of an "additive" specifically excludes micronutrients added to a food for the purpose of fortification, enrichment or restoration) there are no restrictions in so

Table 2. The contribution of fortified products to the intake of vitamin A and vitamin D in EU countries (Modified after [7]). The omission of a country from the Table means that no data are available

Country	Proportional contribution of fortified products to vitamin intake (%) – (m) designates that derived from margarine	
	Vitamin A	Vitamin D
Denmark	11–12 (m)	–
Finland	18–30 (m)	11–47 (m)[a]
Netherlands	25 (m)	60–70 (m)[a]
Norway	15 (m)	48 (m)[a]
Sweden	33	75
United Kindom	14	59

[a] % of total dietary Vitamin D. Cod liver oil *not* included in the figure for Norway and Sweden.

far as the nature of the micronutrients themselves, the foods to which they can be added or the extent of that addition. However, there are specific circumstances where the addition of micronutrients is recommended or compulsory. In the former group is the recommendation that very low calorie diets used in the treatment of obesity should supply the RDA for a full range of vitamins and minerals. In the latter case there are compulsory requirements to add specified micronutrients to flour, bread, margarine and spreadable fats.

The provisions of the Food Safety Act 1990 cover the toxicity aspects of micronutrient addition in that the micronutrient(s) must not be added in such a way as to make the food injurious to health.

It is in the areas of claims made about nutrients as part of product labelling and during advertising that there are strict controls in the United Kingdom particularly so far as health claims are concerned, for example, it is not possible to make medicinal claims describing relationship between a food and a nutrient and the prevention of a disease on food labelling. This is discussed further elsewhere in this book.

In the remainder of the European Community the regulations vary widely from country to country. In France, for example, the addition of vitamins and minerals is strictly controlled and must be justified on the grounds of nutritional needs.

8.7 The Efficacy of the Addition of Micronutrients to Food

There are two approaches to the estimation of the efficacy of addition of micronutrients to the diet. The first, the crudest, would be to use the incidence of certain diseases over the course of a time when additions to the diet were made. It has already been pointed out that attempts to do this for deficiency diseases after the First World War were not successful. In any event it may be that the best approach would be the second, which is to study vulnerable groups within the population rather than the population as a whole.

Much of the supplementation of the diet with micronutrients is probably voluntary through the "over the counter" purchase of vitamins as monotherapy or in combination. It is not clear how much of the individual RDA's this route of intake provides for the population as a whole because quantitative research has not been carried out. There is a strong case for policy relating to the addition of micronutrients to be driven by the relevant science. This is important in view of the rising trend to promote food products using added micronutrients, for example to drinks, biscuits, breakfast cereals marketed at both children and adults. With the prominence of these food products within the supermarkets the consumer may be induced to increase their intake of micronutrients above safe levels. There have been well documented cases of excessive intakes of micronutrients as a consequence of combining food supplements with such products which has been referred to in Chapter 1. The motive behind adding micronutrients to processed foods is partly commercial rather than being wholely nutritional. They add value to products and will therefore enable them to command a higher price. These products are sold at a premium and appeal to those with an interest in their health and diet. These are the consumers that achieve the RNI for micronutrients, exercise regularly and have healthier lifestyles. This pattern has been observed among food supplement users [19]. In the United States research has shown that the enrichment of foods makes a contribution of up to 25% to the intake of iron and a number of vitamins [18]. Given the ubiquitous presence of micronutrients in everyday food sources, it is unlikely that the addition of micronutrients to selected products confers a substantial health benefit to those whose diet is already adequate and excess intake may represent a risk.

8.8 References

1. Corry Mann, H. Rickets: the relative importance of environment and diet as factors of causation. *Medical Research Council, Special report* 1922; No. 68
2. Friend GE. The schoolboy: a study of his nutrition, physical development and health. Cambridge: W Heffer & Sons, Ltd., 1935
3. Drummond J. Scientific approach to food problems during the War. *Nutrition : Dietetics : Catering* 1947; 1: 47–62
4. Woods HF and Bax NDS. Sweetness in the diabetic diet. *Diabetalogia* 1982; 23: 213–215
5. Codex Alimentarius Commission. General Principles for the addition of essential nutrients to foods. *CAC/GLO9* 1987; Codex Alimentarius Vol. 4, Rome
6. Addition of Micronutrients to Food. *The Institute of Food Science & Technology (UK)* 1997; pp 58
7. Scientific considerations for the development of measures on the addition of vitamins and minerals to foodstuffs (1997). SCOOP Task 7.1.1. Working Group P. 101 (Table 2)
8. Guthrie HA. *Introductory nutrition.* St Louis: Times Mirror/Mosby College Publishing, 1986: p. 637
9. Van der Wielen RPJ, Lowik MRH, Van der Berg H. et al. Low 25-hydroxyvitamin D levels among elderly people in Southern Europe. *Lancet* 1995; 346: 207–210
10. Haller J, Lowik M.R.H., Ferry, M., Ferro-Luzit. Nutritional status: blood vitamins A,E, B_6, B_{12}, folic acid and carotene. Euronutrition SENECA investigators. *Eur. J. Clin. Nutr* 1991; 45 (Suppl. 3) 63–82
11. Locksmith GJ and Duff P. Preventing neural tube defects: The importance of periconceptional folic acid supplements. *Obstet.Gynecol* 1998; 91: 1027–1034
12. MRC Vitamin Study Research Group. Prevention of neural tube defects: results of the MRC Vitamin Study. *Lancet* 1991; 338: 132–137
13. Marks J. Vitamin Safety. *Vitamin Information.* Basel: Roche 1989
14. Hathcock JN. Quantitative evaluation of vitamin safety. *Pharmacy Times* May, 1985; 104–113
15. Wald NJ and Bower C. Folic acid, pernicious anaemia and prevention of neural tube defects. *Lancet* 1994; 343: 307
16. D.H.H.S., F.D.A. Food Standards: Amendment of the standards of identity for enriched grain products to require addition of folic acid. Federal Register (1996) 61: 8781–8797
17. Lawrence JM, Petilti DB, Watkins M, Umekubo MA. Trends in serum folate after food fortification. *Lancet* 1999; 354: 915–916
18. Lachance PA, Bauernfeind JC. Concepts and practices of nutrifying foods. In: Bauernfeind JC, Lachance PA, eds. *Nutrient Additions to Food:* Nutritional technological and regulatory aspects. Trumbell, Connecticut: Food and Nutrition Press pp 86, 1991
19. Kirk SFL, Cade JE, Conner MT, Barrett JH. Supplementary issues for women. *BNF Nutrition Bulletin* 1998; 23: 197–202

9 Probiotics and Prebiotics in Health

Colette Shortt, Seppo Salminen, and Marcel Roberfroid

9.1 Introduction

The development of functional foods with the potential to modify gastrointestinal function is currently one of the most promising areas in food science. The gastrointestinal tract is host to about 10^{14} viable bacteria known as the gut flora and much effort has been devoted to defining and characterising the bacteria. It has been known for some time that the gut flora plays a major role in health and that dietary constituents can influence its composition and metabolism. In addition to nutritional and metabolic effects, the gut flora has considerable influence on the immune system. It is thought that gut flora bacteria act as a source of antigens and non-specific immune-modulators. Thus, the identification and characterisation of specific ingredients capable of modulating the composition and/or activity of the gut flora are of particular value in the development of foods for optimum gastrointestinal health.

The ability to target specific health-promoting organisms in the gastrointestinal tract is important both for health maintenance and potentially also of therapeutic value. Both probiotics and prebiotics have been shown to influence the composition and/or activity of specific beneficial bacteria in the gastrointestinal tract. Probiotics are live microbial ingredients that are beneficial to health. Commercially available probiotic preparations consist largely of lactobacilli and/or bifidobacteria although yeasts have also been used. Probiotic bacteria are generally of human origin, safe, can withstand processing conditions and have the ability to survive transit through the gastrointestinal tract. Probiotics can modulate gut flora composition, improve the balance of the gut flora and prevent gut colonisation by specific pathogens. They can also influence bacterial metabolism e.g. enzyme activity and are able to elicit specific systemic and local immune responses.

The prebiotics currently available belong to two key non-digestible carbohydrate groups namely the galacto- and fructo-oligosaccharides. Prebiotic substances are not hydrolysed or absorbed in the small intestine but are available as specific substrates for the gut microflora in the large intestine thus stimulating the growth of one or a small number of the health promoting bacteria. Prebiotics thus modulate the gut microflora, but they also improve stool bulking, improve calcium absorption in the colon and, in experimental models, they inhibit the development of aberrant crypt foci and adenomas in the colon. They are also classified as dietary fibre. An approach involving both pre- and probiotics – the synbiotic approach – is one which may have the potential to extend product shelf-life, improve viability and survival of probiotic strains and enhance the stimulation of selected beneficial species. The role of probiotics and prebiotics in the maintenance of gastrointestinal health and potential reduction of risk factors will be discussed in Sects. 9.2 and 9.3.

9.2 Probiotic Bacteria in Human Health: An Overview

Colette Shortt and Seppo Salminen

9.2.1 Introduction

A probiotic is a live microbial food ingredient that beneficially influences human health [1, 2]. Probiotics have been used historically in different cultures for the treatment of gastroenteritis in children and adults in the form of fermented dairy foods, fermented vegetables and fermented cereals [3]. Probiotics act within the gastrointestinal tract (GIT) and health effects have been reported within the oral cavity, stomach, small intestine, and large intestine. Probiotics mainly consist of Lactic acid bacteria (LAB), but also bifidobacteria and yeast have been successfully used and other types of microbes are under investigation.

Probiotic studies have been conducted in animals and humans and some species specificity has been reported. One of the major tasks has been defining the strains and conducting good clinical studies to clearly document the health effects and their mechanisms. Today specific probiotic strains are available with scientifically proven health benefits for humans. New strains and functional food products based on these strains are likely to emerge with effects in the areas of GIT health maintenance, disease risk-reduction and prevention of gastrointestinal diseases.

9.2.2 Probiotics and Dietary Modulation

While many are aware that there are 10^{13} cells in the human body most of us are unaware that the human body is also host to 10^{14} bacteria. The majority of which are found in the GIT and are known as the gut microflora [4, 5]. The bacteria comprising the gut microflora are estimated to weigh ~ 1 kg and include several hundred cultured species of bacteria. There are many more species that are unculturable by the available traditional methods.

The gut microflora is acquired rapidly during and shortly after birth. At first *E. coli* and *Streptococcus* species predominate, but in breast-fed infants there is a sharp increase in the number of bifidobacteria with a concomitant decrease in *E. coli* and *Streptococcus* [6]. Generally after weaning, streptococci and *E. coli* populations decrease and by the second year of life an adult-type flora has been established. The method of birth has a profound effect on the gut microflora development. Infants born by caesarean section tend to have a simple gut microflora which develops slowly during the first 6 months compared to that of infants born by the normal method of delivery who tend to have a more diverse microflora resulting from contact with the mother's birth canal [7].

Bacterial numbers and composition vary considerably along the GIT. The density of microorganisms in the gut microflora increases dramatically from less than 10^3/g in the stomach due to the harsh acidic conditions to greater than 10^{10}/g in the large intestine (Table 1) [4, 5, 8]. The reported concentrations also depend on the method of enumeration of bacteria. The growth and metabolic activity of the gut microflora have a tremendous influence on our physiological and nutritional wellbeing. It has even been suggested that the metabolic activity of the gut microflora is potentially greater than that of the liver. The gut microflora therefore plays an important role in the maintenance of health: forming a healthy gut barrier, stimulating the immune system, protecting the host from invading bacteria and viruses, and aiding digestion [4–6].

While many of the bacterial species that comprise the gut microflora exert beneficial effects, some, in certain circumstances, have the potential to exert harmful effects e.g. Clostridia, sulfate reducers and amino-acid-fermenting species [6, 8]. An optimum gut microflora balance is one in which beneficial bacteria, such as the Gram-positive lactobacilli and bifidobacteria predominate over potentially harmful bacteria [9, 10]. Many factors, such as diet composition, antibiotic therapy, infections, food poisoning, environment, stress, health status and ageing can influence the balance of the gut flora [6, 11].

The concept of ingesting live bacteria as a means of modulating the gut flora to maintain health and promote beneficial effects is not new. At the beginning

Table 1. Type and concentration of bacteria in the human large intestine [8]

Bacteria	Concentration (mean and range) Log_{10}/g dry wt of faeces
Bacteroides	11.3 (9.2–13.5)
Eubacteria	10.7 (5.0–13.3)
Bifidobacteria	10.2 (4.9–13.4)
Clostridia	9.8 (3.3–13.1)
Lactiobacilli	9.6 (3.6–12.5)
Ruminococci	10.2 (4.6–12.8)
Peptostreptococci	10.1 (3.8–12.6)
Peptococci	10.0 (5.1–12.9)
Methanobrevivbacter	8.8 (7.0–10.5)
Desulfovibrio	8.4 (5.2–10.9)
Propionibacteria	9.4 (4.3–12.0)
Actinomyces	9.2 (5.7–11.1)
Streptococci	8.9 (3.9–12.9)
Fusobacteria	8.4 (5.1–11.0)
Escherichia	8.6 (3.9–12.3)

of the 20th Century, the Nobel laureate Elie Metchnikoff was the first to propose a scientific rationale for the beneficial effects of the bacteria in yoghurt. In his book *The Prolongation of Life* he postulated that yoghurt consumption played a role in health and he attributed the long life of Bulgarian peasants to their intake of yoghurt containing *Lactobacillus* species [12]. Tissier in 1906 advocated the administration of bifidobacteria to infants suffering from diarrhoea in the belief that the bifidobacteria displaced the pathogenic bacteria [13]. In Japan in the early 1930s Shirota focused his research on selecting beneficial strains of LAB that could survive passage through the gut and on the use of such strains to develop fermented milk drinks [14]. More recently, Gorbach and Goldin isolated a probiotic strain that survives the gastric conditions, tolerates bile acids, adheres to intestinal cells and leads to specific health benefits [15].

9.2.3 Concept of Probiotic Bacteria

The word probiotic is derived from the Greek meaning 'for life' and the definition of probiotics has evolved since the early 1960s. The word was used to describe substances produced by one protozoan to stimulate the growth of another; tissue extracts that stimulated microbial growth and animal feed supplements including organisms and substances that had a beneficial effect on an animal by contributing to its intestinal flora balance [16]. In 1989, Fuller defined a probiotic as 'a live microbial feed supplement, which beneficially affects the host animal by improving its intestinal microbial balance' by increasing health-promoting bacterial groups [17]. This definition stressed the importance of live cells as a component of an effective probiotic. Two years later Huis in't Veld & Havenaar redefined and expanded the definition to 'a mono- or mixed culture of live microorganisms which applied to man or animal affects beneficially the host by improving the properties of the indigenous microflora' [18]. This definition developed the concept of probiotics in several ways:

- it introduced the concept of human use
- probiotic activity is not restricted to the gut microflora but includes the possible application to microbial communities at other sites e.g. respiratory tract, urogenital tract, skin
- the probiotic may consist of a mono-culture or a cocktail of cultures.

Recently a group of European scientists, as part of an EU-supported concerted action project, suggested that probiotics for use in human nutrition are best defined as 'live microbial food ingredients that are beneficial to health' [2]. This definition taking into account results from recent research allows for the possibility of non-microflora mediated probiotic effects e.g. direct probiotic effects on the immune system.

9.2.4 Selection of Probiotic Strains

In selecting probiotic bacteria for use in human foods, certain criteria as outlined in Table 2 are followed [19, 20]. Probiotic bacteria used in foods for human consumption are generally of human origin and are non-pathogenic. In addition, they retain significant viability during processing and transit through the gut [19]. Probiotics are predominantly LAB though not exclusively, e.g. *S. boulardii* is a probiotic yeast. Examples of probiotic strains are given in Table 3.

Validated in vitro models are available that allow rapid screening of potential probiotic bacteria [21]. It is also possible to monitor the kinetics of transit of probiotic bacteria through the GIT using DNA-based technologies and a variety of techniques based on the polymerase chain reaction [6]. Many critics of probiotics question whether probiotic strains remain viable during GIT transit. However, there are many studies using classical microbiological techniques and more sophisticated DNA-based techniques confirming that selected probiotic strains remain viable after transit through the GIT [22–27]. Following ingestion of a food containing probiotic bacteria, there is an increase in the count of the probiotic bacteria, which decreases once consumption has ceased i.e., there is a transient colonisation (see Fig. 1).

Several studies have evaluated the effect of varying doses of specific probiotic strains on faecal microbial changes. Daily administration of *Lactobacillus*

Table 2. Selection criteria for selecting a probiotic bacteria

Human origin
Non-pathogenic
Acid & bile tolerant
Ability to withstand technological processes and remain viable during shelf-life period
Adherence to intestinal mucosa (mucus or mucosal cells) may be used for specific uses
Evidence of potential beneficial effects

Table 3. Microorganisms used in probiotic products around the world

Lactobacilli	Bifidobacteria	Other LAB	Non-LAB
L. acidophilus	*B. animalis*	*E. faecium*	*B. cereus*
L. casei	*B. breve*	*E. faecalis*	*E. coli*
L. johnsonii	*B. infantis*		*S. boulardii*
L. reuteri	*B. longum*		*Cl. butyricum*
L. rhamnosus	*B. adolescentis*		
L. salvarius	*B. lactis*		
L. crispatus			

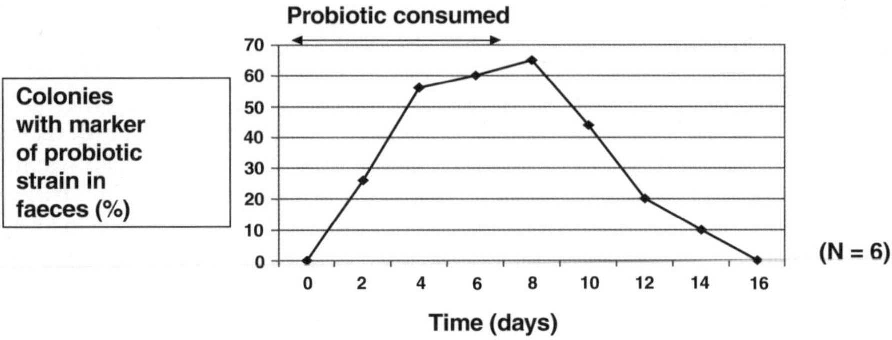

Fig. 1. Appearance of ingested probiotic bacteria in faeces [22]

casei Shirota at levels from 6.5×10^9 to 3×10^{10} have been shown to lead to substantial increases in the number of faecal LcS [14]. It has also been shown that to achieve faecal recovery of *Lactobacillus* GG (LGG) the lowest level of this strain which must be administered is 1×10^{10} cfu/d when given as a freeze-dried powder. The dose required for recovery can be lower if a protective enterosoluble coating encapsulates the strain. When the strain is administered in a fermented milk 1.2×10^{10} cfu/d is effective in achieving a significant increase in mean faecal LGG content [28].

The mechanism(s) of action of probiotic bacteria in promoting health include the following: adherence to intestinal mucosa and mucus, production of anti-microbial substances, antagonism against pathogens, competition for adhesion sites (competitive exclusion), interaction with gut associated lymphoid tissue (GALT), immune-regulation, in-activation of harmful components within the intestinal contents (binding of toxins), regulation of the metabolic activity of the intestinal microflora and overall normalisation of the intestinal microflora [20, 26]. Most reported health effects are based on the above mentioned mechanisms and these are referred to in Table 4.

Some of the established and recent entries into the probiotic market are illustrated in Table 5. There has been some criticism regarding the composition and labelling of some probiotic products [30–32]. Generally, the criticism is targeted at probiotic supplements that have been shown, albeit using limited samples, to either not contain the number or type of bacteria stated on the labels or to contain strains not mentioned on the labels. Probiotic yoghurts and fermented milks have generally received favourable reviews when tested [32]. However, this highlights the importance of rigorous quality control and assurance in the manufacture of probiotic products in maintaining and building consumer confidence.

It cannot be assumed that all probiotic strains from even a specific species have the same or even any desirable properties. It is important to choose products that provide details of the strain(s) and ensure the stability of the probiotic strains or indicate the total viable count of organisms present in the product [33]. It is also important to follow the manufacturers' instructions regarding the amount (g or ml) to consume. For gut health maintenance probiotic products

Table 4. Reported studies and effects of currently available probiotics [2, 29]

Strain	Reported effect in clinical studies	Scientifically established effects[a]
Lactobacillus johnsonii LJ1	Adherence to human intestinal cells, balances intestinal microflora, immune enhancement, adjuvant in *Helicobacter pylori* treatment	Adherence, immune enhancement
Lactobacillus acidophilus NCFB 1748	Lowering of faecal enzyme activity, decreasing faecal mutagenicity, prevention of radiotherapy- related diarrhoea, improvement of constipation	Decreasing mutagenicity, alleviates constipation
Lactobacillus GG (ATCC 53013)	Prevention of antibiotic associated diarrhoea, treatment and prevention of rotavirus diarrhoea, treatment of relapsing *Clostridium difficile* diarrhoea, prevention of acute diarrhoea, stabilisation of Crohn's disease, antagonistic against cariogenic bacteria	Shortening of rotavirus diarrhoea, increase in bifidobacteria, prevention/ and treatment of antibiotic associated diarrhoea
Lactobacillus acidophilus NFCM	Lowering of faecal enzyme activity, high lactase activity, treatment of lactose intolerance, production of bacteriocins	Alleviation of symptoms of lactose intolerance
Lactobacillus casei Shirota	Prevention of intestinal disturbances, balancing intestinal bacteria, lowering faecal enzyme activities, positive effects on superficial bladder cancer	Immune enhancement, prevention of recurrence of superficial bladder cancer, Normalisation of the intestinal microflora
Streptococcus thermophilus;	No effect on rotavirus diarrhoea, no immune enhancing effect during rotavirus diarrhoea, no effect on faecal enzymes	Alleviation of symptoms of lactose intolerance
Lactobacillus bulgaricus	Treatment of viral diarrhoea including rotavirus diarrhoea, balancing intestinal microflora	Prevention of rotavirus diarrhoea
Bifidobacterium lactis	Faecal enzyme reduction, survival in the intestinal tract	Altering intestinal metabolic activity
Lactobacillus gasseri (ADH)	Colonizing the intestinal tract	Shortening of rotavirus diarrhoea
Lactobacillus reuteri	Mainly animal studies- possibly an emerging human probiotic	Prevention of antibiotic associated diarrhoea, treatment of *Clostridium difficile* colitis
Saccharomyces boulardi	Prevention of antibiotic associated diarrhoea, treatment *of Clostridium difficile* colitis	

[a] Proven by at least two published independently conducted clinical studies in humans.

Table 5. Food products containing probiotic bacteria

Product	Company
Actimel	Danone
Fysiq	Campina Melkunie
Gefilus	Valio
LA-7 plus	Bauer
LC1	Nestle
Mil Mil	Yakult
ProCult 3	Muller
Proviva	Skånemeijerier,
Rela	Ingman Foods
SynBalance	Toni Lait
Vifit	Campina Melkunie
Yakult	Yakult
Yosa	Bioferme

with concentrations in the region of 10^8 cfu/ml or greater are generally recommended by manufacturers. While supplements are convenient for delivering high or biotherapeutic concentrations of probiotic bacteria, there is some evidence to suggest that compliance may not be optimal with supplements. Probiotic foods e.g. fermented dairy products, juices, oatmeal gruels in addition to providing high stable concentrations of probiotic bacteria are also excellent sources of nutrients and can easily be incorporated into a balanced diet. Modern processing allows for the production of excellent tasting fermented products with high counts of probiotic bacteria which are guaranteed over the shelf-life period e.g. a new probiotic fermented milk on the Japanese market contains 40×10^9 cfu per bottle.

Safety issues relating to new probiotics should be assessed according to the EU novel food regulations. The use of LAB in foods has a long history and most strains are considered commensal microorganisms with no pathogenic potential. Their ubiquitous presence in the human GIT together with their traditional use in fermented foods and dairy products without significant problems attest to their safety [34]. Members of the genus *Lactobacillus* are most commonly given safe or generally recognised as safe (GRAS) status. Members of the genera *Streptococcus* and *Enterococcus* may contain opportunistic pathogens.

The safety of probiotics has been assessed in recent reviews and clinical reports have drawn attention to a few cases of human bacteraemia associated with the presence of LAB. A variety of strains of probiotic organisms have been used in the clinical treatment of gastrointestinal disorders and in the prevention of gut colonisation by pathogens in both children and adults [29]. These have included conditions where mucosal integrity was impaired by antibiotics, radiotherapy or acute diarrhoea of bacterial or viral origin. No evidence of opportunistic infections or other ill-effects by probiotics have been observed in these studies. In addition, animal studies indicate an absence of infectivity and specific toxicity studies show no sign of toxic or harmful effects even at extremely high dose levels. Generally, established probiotics are considered safe [34, 35].

Aspects of the safety of probiotic bacteria can be studied using *in vitro* methods, animal models and human subjects. Some recommendations are given in the review of an European Demonstration project work [36]. Two recent Finnish studies confirm that the number of infections associated with LAB is extremely small [37, 38]. However, epidemiological surveillance has been suggested as an additional safety measure for future probiotics.

9.2.5 Conclusion

Both the efficacy of probiotics for a given health effect and the safety of the strain in its intended use have to be documented in well-designed studies. For efficacy, these should be hypothesis-based human studies as proposed by the International Life Science Institute Europe working group [1, 2]. Such studies should focus on specific health effects with established biomarkers and be conducted according to the guidelines set for good clinical studies. In a recent European scientific assessment of functional foods it was concluded that certain health effects of probiotic bacteria can be considered scientifically proven for specific strains [1, 2]. The criterion for scientifically proven was that the effect was established in at least two good independent human studies. The effects of probiotics can be divided into two groups: effects reported in scientific literature and effects scientifically established in at least two human studies with supporting information from *in vitro* studies and animal studies (Tables 4 and 6).

Some of the potential health effects of probiotics have been highlighted in this chapter and the current status of research is healthy in its diversity with many well-characterised probiotic strains being used in well-designed human studies [39–41]. It is clear that there are many medical conditions being investigated for which probiotic therapy or the reduction in the risk of diseases may hold some promise [42, 43]. Such areas include inflammatory bowel disease (Crohn's, Ulcerative colitis, Pouchitis), food allergy, oral rehydration therapy, superficial bladder cancer, urogenital infections [42]. Research efforts worldwide are now focusing on the development of probiotic products containing bacteria selected for their specific health-enhancing characteristics.

Table 6. Scientifically established health effects of probiotics [2]

Established effects in humans	Reduction of the duration of rotavirus diarrhoea
	Alleviation of the symptoms of lactose intolerance Prevention of the recurrence of superficial bladder tumours Decreasing faecal bacterial enzyme activity Decreasing faecal mutagenicity Immune enhancement

9.3 Prebiotics in Human Health: An Overview

Marcel Roberfroid

9.3.1 Introduction

A prebiotic has been defined as "a non-digestible food ingredient that beneficially affects the host by selectively stimulating the growth and/or activity of one or a limited number of bacteria in the colon" [9]. This concept implies that some dietary components resist the hydrolysis by the digestive enzymes and/or are not absorbed in the upper part of the gastro-intestinal tract including the small intestine. Indeed, these compounds must pass into the large bowel where most of the indigenous intestinal microflora are located. A wide variety of dietary carbohydrates, especially resistant starch, dietary fibres and non-digestible oligosaccharides have such characteristics and they provide available substrates for bacterial fermentation in the colon. The colonic fermentation of such "malabsorbed", "non-digestible", or "resistant" carbohydrates (poly- and oligosaccharides) plays a role in salvaging part of their energy, in controlling transit time, stool bulking and stool frequency, in influencing nutrient, especially mineral, bioavailability, in producing short chain fatty acids that are known to play physiological roles such as control of mucosal motility and epithelial cell proliferation or in modulating immune activity and endocrine functions [46]. But prebiotics are more than "malabsorbed", "non-digestible", or "resistant" carbohydrates because, when they reach the large bowel, they have a specific metabolism therein – directed towards advantageous rather than adverse bacteria. This would ultimately lead to a marked change in the colonic microflora composition e.g. by selectively stimulating the growth of bacteria like the *Bifidobacteria* that are generally recognized as being beneficial for health. The most efficient prebiotics, will also reduce numbers and activities of potentially pathogenic organisms. But since the gut content is not really accessible, in humans, for microbiological analysis, faecal microflora is used as a surrogate marker and the prebiotic effect is demonstrated by showing changes in the composition of the faecal microflora.

9.3.2 The Prebiotics

At present, food components for which a prebiotic effect has been reported are the non-digestible oligosaccharides (NDO) [47]. The NDOs contain mixtures of oligomers of different chain lengths and are characterised by the average number of osyl (like glucose, fructose, galactose or xylose) moieties, referred to as the degree of polymerisation (DP). As discussed recently [48], there is no rational physiological or chemical reason for discriminating oligosaccharides and polysaccharides on the basis of DP.

NDOs are oligomeric carbohydrates, the osidic bond of which is in a spatial configuration that allows resistance to hydrolytic activities of intestinal digestive enzymes. But they are fermented by, at least some of, the colonic bacteria. This fermentation produces short chain fatty acids and gases as well as increased metabolic energy, growth and proliferation of these bacteria. NDOs for which, at least some, data have been published to support a prebiotic effect are listed in Table 7.

Currently, there are little comparative data on the relative efficiencies of these potentially prebiotic oligosaccharides, or on their selectivity at a species, or even genus, level. It is often the case that a prebiotic effect is levelled against certain NDOs, or other dietary carbohydrates, without a full and careful investigation of their fermentation profile. It is indeed critical that as many components of the faecal microbiota as possible are measured. These should at least include bacteroides, *bifidobacteria*, clostridia, Gram positive cocci, coliforms, lactobacilli, total aerobes and total anaerobes. Simple stimulation of growth of bifidobacteria and/or lactobacilli is insufficient to substantiate a prebiotic property without determining effects on other faecal microorganisms – as it is the **selectivity** of effect that determines classification as a prebiotic. Clearly, studies using pure bacterial cultures are of very limited, if any, value in this respect, unless they are also supported by mixed culture work. But the ultimate proof must come from in vivo human studies where faecal samples, which have been collected and stored correctly, are analysed for their composition in terms of different bacteria. These bacteria should be further well characterised using either classical culture combined with a conventional microbiological approach towards identification and/or modern molecular genotyping methods. Indeed, it is the effect of the NDO in a **competitive** ecological environment that is key [61].

Among the malabsorbed oligosaccharides, those composed primarily of fructose occupy a leading position in food science. Fructooligosaccharide is

Table 7. Non-digestible oligosaccharides for which at least some, data have been published to support a prebiotic effect [49]

Oligosaccharides	References
Inulin-type fructans or	[50, 51]
Fructooligosaccharides (FOS)	[52, 53]
Soybean oligosaccharides (raffinose and stachyose)	
Galactooligosaccharides or Trans galactooligosaccharides (TOS)	[54–56]
Galactosylsucrose	[57]
Isomaltooligosaccharides	[58]
Palatinose condensates	[59]
Xylooligosaccharides	[60]

used as a generic name for all malabsorbed oligosaccharides composed mainly of fructose. Strictly from the point of view of nomenclature, these molecules are "inulin-type fructans", the linear β-(2–1)-fructans which are different from the "levans", the β-(2–6), often branched, fructans [50]. Inulin-type fructans are by far the most extensively studied compounds and are clear 'market leader' prebiotics.

The inulin-type fructans are composed of β-D-fructofuranoses attached by β-2–1 linkages. The first monomer of the chain is either a α-D-glucopyranosyl or β-D-fructopyranosyl residue. They constitute a series of homologous oligosaccharides derived from sucrose and represented by the formula GF_n or FF_n. The natural NDOs which are extracted from chicory roots (*Cichorium intybus*) are a mixture of either GF_n (α-D glucopyranosyl-[β-D furanosyl]n_{-1}-D fructofuranoside) or $GF_n + FF_n$ (β-D fructopyranosyl-[β-D fructofuranosyl]$_{n-1}$-D fructofuranoside) molecules, with the number of fructose units varying from 2 to 60–65 units. As food ingredients [62] they are available as native inulin (inulin ST or standard, average DP = 10) and high molecular weight inulin (inulin HP or high performance, average DP = 20), enzymatically-hydrolysed inulin (oligofructose, average DP = 4) and a mixture of inulin HP and oligofructose (synergy 1), all of which occur naturally in miscellaneous edible plants such as garlic, onion, asparagus, artichoke, banana and, wheat [63].

The average daily intake of inulin-type fructans varies from 1 up to 12 g depending on dietary habits [63, 64]. Oligofructose can also be produced by enzymatic conversion of sucrose to give a mixture of GF_2, GF_3, GF_4 (with an DP = 3.8), sucrose, glucose and fructose.

A potentially important class of prebiotics are the galactooligosaccharides or transgalactooligosaccharides which are produced industrially from lactose by transglycolsylation reactions and consist of galactosyl derivatives of lactose with β-1–3 and β-1–6 linkages.

The purported prebiotic nature of fructooligosaccharides and galactooligosaccharides are explainable, at least in part, by the linkage-specificity of the *Bifidobacterium* β-fructosidase and β-galactosidase respectively. These enzymes are cell-bound [65, 66].

Glucose-based maltooligosaccharides and xylooligosaccharides are candidate prebiotics. However, specific enzymes for the degradation of these molecules have not yet been identified.

9.3.3 Malabsorption of the Non-Digestible Oligosaccharides

The β-configuration of the anomeric C_2 in their fructose monomers makes inulin-type fructans resistant to the hydrolysis by human digestive enzymes (α-glucosidase; maltase-isomaltase; sucrase) which are mostly specific for α-osidic linkages. In normal physiological conditions they also resist the acid hydrolysis in the stomach. The most convincing data have been obtained in human intervention studies with ileostomy volunteers. These studies show that 86–88% of the ingested dose (10–30 g) of inulin or oligofructose are recovered in the ileostomy effluent supporting the conclusion that these carbohydrates are practically undigestible in the small intestine of man [67, 68]. Using an intubation technique in human volunteers, Molis et al. [69] have similarly concluded that fructooligosaccharides are malabsorbed in the human small intestine (89% recovery). The small but still significant loss of fructooligosaccharides in the upper part of the gastrointestinal tract could be due to fermentation by the microbial population colonizing the ileum especially in ileostomy patients [67] and/or to hydrolysis of the lowest molecular weight oligomers [69]. In their recent review on the malabsorption characteristics of inulin-type fructans, Andersson et al. have concluded that "inulin and oligofructose pass through the small bowel without degradation and (furthermore) without influencing the absorption of nutrients and minerals especially calcium, magnesium, and iron Ca, Mg and Fe" [70].

Published data on the resistance of other oligosaccharides to digestion in the upper gastrointestinal tract are less available than for the inulin-type fructans. Predominantly the available evidence comes from in vitro experiments or is based on hydrogen production and exhalation or on stimulation of growth of specific faecal microorganisms in animal models. No in-vivo human data are available yet.

Thus, the non-digestibility of isomaltooligosaccharides, soybean oligosaccharides, galactooligosaccharides, palatinose condensates or xylooligosacchairdes remain to be convincingly demonstrated.

9.3.4 Fermentation in the Large Bowel: The Prebiotic Effect

The large bowel is by far the most heavily colonized segment of the gastrointestinal tract, with up to 10^{12} (mostly anaerobic) bacteria/g of gut content. These bacteria belong to a wide variety of genera, species and strains. Through the process of fermentation, these colonic bacteria produce a wide variety of metabolites and salvage part of the energy from the malabsorbed food components in particular carbohydrates. Among these metabolites are the short chain fatty acids that serve to salvage part of the energy of the malabsorbed food components especially malabsorbed carbohydrates and which play systemic physiological roles.

Evidence for the fermentation of inulin-type fructans by bacteria colonizing the large bowel has come both from in vitro and in vivo studies that have recently been reviewed and evaluated [51]. At nutritional doses (up to 20–40 g/day) these malabsorbed carbohydrates are quantitatively fermented and not excreted in the faeces and they are metabolized to produce short chain fatty acids mainly acetate, butyrate and propionate.

As compared to most other malabsorbed carbohydrates (e.g. resistant starch and dietary fibres), the colonic fermentation of inulin-type fructans is accompanied by a significant change in the composition of the colonic microbiota due to selective proliferation of bifidobacteria and a concomitant reduction in the number of other bacteria like bacteroides, fusobacteria or clostridia. Based on the results of well designed human studies that have shown significant changes in the composition of human faecal flora it can be concluded that inulin-type fructans (3–15 g/day for a few weeks) are prebiotic [51,71,72]. But, even though some studies showed a significant reduction in the number of clostridia, the health benefit(s) (e.g. reducing the risk of intestinal infections) of such a change in the compostion of the colonic microbiota still need to be established. A recent report by Hunter et al. has shown that, at a daily dose of 6 g (3 × 2 g), oligofructose had no therapeutic value in patients with irritable bowel syndrome [73]. But, in an experimental model of necrotising enterocolitis in quails, Catala et al. have reported data that support the hypothesis that oligofructose might prevent the overgrowth of bacteria known to play a role in this pathology in preterm neonates [74].

For other NDOs, in vivo studies have also been performed with doses ranging from 3 g up to 15 g/d, given for 1, 2 or 3 week periods. For soybean oligosaccharides, a dose of 10 g given twice daily for 3 weeks, significantly increased the number of bifidobacteria whilst slightly decreasing clostridia counts [52]. A dose of 3 g/d not only increased bifidobacteria but also bacteroides and eubacteria [53]. For the galactooligosaccharides, Tanaka et al. [54] and Ito et al. [55,56] have reported an increase both in bifidobacteria and lactobacilli for doses ranging from 3 to 10 g/d. A daily dose of galactosylsucrose (5 or 10 g/d) similarly stimulated the growth of bifidobacteria after 1 and 2 weeks of ingestion [57]. An isomaltooligosaccharide dose of 13.5 g/d for 2 weeks significantly increased bifidobacteria both in adult and elderly volunteers [58]. Palatinose condensate may also stimulate the growth of bifidobacteria [59]. For all these NDOs, except galactooligosaccharides, only a single human intervention study has been performed that needs to be repeated before any prebiotic effect can be claimed. Moreover, as discussed above, great care should be given to quantify the faecal microflora and to identify changes in its composition.

9.3.5 Physiological Effects in the Gastro-Intestinal Tract

The fermentation of NDOs in the colon has a series of consequences that affect large bowel physiology. Firstly it produces short chain fatty acids that create a more acidic environment that is beneficial for the development of bacteria like bifidobacteria or lactobacilli but is detrimental to the growth of potentially pathogenic species like clostridia or *Escherichia coli*. Furthermore, in this acidic environment ammonia and amines become protonated and are thus much less absorbable and more readily excretable. Secondly, it leads to a proliferation of colonic bacteria resulting in an increase in faecal mass and consequently a beneficial bulking effect. As a consequence of these two large bowel processes (i.e. production of acids and proliferation of bacteria), only part of the energy of the malabsorbed oligosaccharides is salvaged. As compared to absorbed carbohydrates (e.g. starch or sucrose) NDOs have thus a lower energy value for the host. Caloric values between 1 and 2.1 Kcal/g or 25 to 50% of the caloric value of sucrose have been reported especially for inulin-type fructans [75]. But, as stated recently by a group of experts, 'all carbohydrates which are more or less completely fermented in human colon, should be given a caloric value of 1.5 Kcal/g (6.3 KJ/g)' [48]. Indeed the daily intake of these dietary carbohydrates is likely to remain small, probably often not more than 5% of total daily calorie intake. It is thus not justifiable to spend too much effort in trying to give, for such carbohydrate, a precise calorie value, the determination of which will depend on the protocol used and, probably also, on the diet in which they are included.

An other physiological consequence of the consumption of NDOs that has been recently reported for the inulin-type fructans is an increase bioavailability of calcium. Such an effect has extensively been studied in rat and hamster [76–78]. These studies have led to conclude that, most probably because of their malabsorption and their colonic fermentation, these food ingredients facilitate calcium absorption from the large bowel compartment thus complementing the process that takes place in the small bowel. Change in colonic pH, production of short chain fatty acids, and increase in mucosal concentration of the calbinding protein in the colon have been proposed as hypotheses to explain that effect. Besides increased calcium bioavailability, it has also been shown both in rat and in hamster that feeding fructooligosaccharides increase calcium concentration and improve bone structure [77, 78]. More recently, two human trials (one in adolescents and one in adults) have shown that supplementing the diet with either 15 g oligofructose [79] or 40 g of inulin [80] significantly increases the apparent absorption of calcium by 12% and 11% respectively. The first study used the calcium balance measurement whereas the second utilized the double stable isotope technique. The result of the first study has recently been confirmed using 8 g/d of "synergy 1" (a mixture of oligofructose and high molecular weight inulin) [Abrams S, personal communication].

Nevertheless and besides their prebiotic effect, NDOs, because they are malabsorbed and fermented in the colon, are part of the dietary fibre complex [81]. In particular it has been shown that inulin-type fructans have a faecal bulking effect that is comparable to that of a soluble fibre like pectin [8]. Moreover, an internationally validated method derived from the AOAC method for dietary fibre analysis exists to quantify inulin and oligofructose in plants and food products [82]. For the purpose of food labeling they are classified as dietary fibre.

9.3.6 Prebiotics and the Risk of Colon Cancer

Over the last two years, reports have been published that repeatedly demonstrated that feeding inulin-type fructans to rats previously treated with a colon carcinogen (i.e. dimethylhydrazine or azoxymethane) reduces the incidence of the so-called aberrant crypt foci in the colon [83, 84]. In one of these studies, the synbiotic approach that combines oligofructose (prebiotic) and bifidobacteria (probiotic) was reported to be more active than either the prebiotic or the probiotic alone [84]. Furthermore, Pierre et al. [85] have demonstrated that oligofructose reduces or even suppresses the number of tumors and stimulates the gut associated lymphoid tissue, as measured by the number of lymphoid nodules in transgenic *Min* mice. Even though still experimental, these data suggest that inulin-type fructans might play a role in reducing the risk of developing preneoplastic lesions in the colon. Moreover such an effect might not be limited to inulin-type fructans. Indeed, as discussed by Rumney and Rowland [86] 'non-digestible oligosaccharides may exert anti-carcinogenic effects firstly because they have been shown to beneficially affect certain biomarkers known to be associated with cancer risk (e.g. reduction of bacterial β-glucuronidase and nitrate reductase activity, pH, and conversion of a dietary carcinogen to its genotoxic metabolite in caecal contents or faeces of NDOs fed rats and human volunteers respectively) and secondly because they stimulate the growth of lactic acid bacteria for which evidence of anti-genotoxic and anti-carcinogenic effects have been reported'.

9.3.7 Conclusion: Prebiotics, What Benefit(s) for Human Health?

Prebiotics have nutritional properties which, in the present state of knowledge, originate mainly in resistance to the hydrolytic activities in the upper part of the gastro-intestinal tract of monogastric organisms followed by extensive fermentation in the large bowel leading to significant changes in the composition of the colonic microbiota. The gastrointestinal target functions which are associated with a balanced microflora together with an optimal gut associated lymphoid tissue (GALT) are relevant to the state of well-being and health and to the reduction of the risk of diseases. The colonic microflora is a complex ecosystem the functions of which are a consequence of the combined action of the microbes that, besides interacting with the GALT, contribute to salvage of nutrient energy and produce end-metabolic products like the short chain fatty acids (SCFAs) that play a role in cell differentiation, cell proliferation and metabolic regulatory processes. It is generally assumed that the group of potentially health promoting bacteria includes principally bifidobacteria, lactobacilli and bacteroides which are and possibly should remain the most important genera in humans. Changes in the composition of the faecal flora, a recognised surrogate marker of the residual colonic microbiota, can be considered as a marker, both indicator and factor, of large bowel functions. They might play a role in gastrointestinal infections and diarrhoea, constipation, irritable bowel syndrome, inflammatory bowel diseases and colorectal cancer.

Probiotics (e.g. lactobacilli or bifidobacteria) and prebiotics (like chicory inulin and its hydrolysate oligofructose) and synbiotics (a combination of both pro- and prebiotics) are recent concepts in nutrition that have already and will in the future be used to support the development of functional foods targeted towards gut functions. Their effects may include:

- stimulation of the activity of the GALT (eg increased IgA response, production of cytokines...),
- reduction of the duration of episodes of rotavirus infection,
- change in the composition of the faecal flora to reach/maintain a composition in which bifidobacteria and/or lactobacilli become predominant in number, a situation that is considered optimal,
- increase in faecal mass (stool bulking) and stool frequency,
- increase in calcium bioavailability via colonic absorption (e.g. inulin).

By reference to the recently released European consensus on scientific concepts of functional foods [1], prebiotics, especially inulin-type fructans (but also synbiotics) are thus good candidates to be recognised as functional food ingredients for which claims should become authorized [87]. Such claims should relate to enhanced gastrointestinal functions (e.g. composition of colonic flora, bulking effect, and bowel habit and, calcium bioavailability...) or risk of developing a disease such as colon cancer. In addition animal data show that feeding inulin-type fructans significantly reduces hepatic lipogenesis and triglyceridemia [88, 89]. But so far, trials that have evaluated their effect on lipid parameters in humans have produced contradictory results [90–92]. More work is thus still needed especially in performing human nutrition studies, but sound hypotheses have already been formulated that fully justify these studies. All these aspects of the nutritional properties of non-digestible oligosaccharides have been critically evaluated by a group of European experts who have published their consensus views on the topic [93].

9.3.8 Conclusions

The gastrointestinal functions that are associated with a balanced intestinal microflora together with an optimal gut associated lymphoid tissue system are relevant to the maintenance of health and well-being and also contribute to the reduction of risk of disease.

Probiotics: Evidence suggests that probiotics can re-inforce the normal gut flora and contribute to the maintenance of an optimum gut flora balance which is conducive to health. In particular, they can restore gut microflora balance after disruption e.g. after antibiotic therapy or a bout of travellers' diarrhoea. Probiotics can also aid specific digestive functions e.g. alleviating the effects of lactose intolerance, decreasing mutagenic activity in the gut by lowering the activities of microbial enzyme which may play a role in carcinogenesis. Specific probiotics have been used effectively to shorten the duration of rotavirus diarrhoea, in the treatment of food-related allergic dermatitis and to alleviate the symptoms of irritable bowel syndrome. Recent preliminary research also suggests that probiotic therapy may play a role in the management of inflammatory bowel disease and in the suppression of *H. pylori*.

Prebiotics: Being part of the dietary fibre complex they share many of the effects of dietary fibre such as, production of short chain fatty acids mainly acetate, butyrate and propionate, reduction in colonic pH and increase in faecal weight. In addition, they selectively encourage bifidobacteria proliferation with a concomitant reduction in potentially pathogenic bacteria. The health benefits associated with these changes though not well established are increasing. For example the bulking effects lead to dilution of carcinogens and more rapid intestinal transit which may contribute to reducing the risk of preneoplastic lesion development in the colon. Research also suggests that prebiotics may play a role in the prevention of gastrointestinal infections, shortening of the duration of diarrhoea, alleviation of the symptoms of irritable bowel syndrome and contribute to decreasing the risk of developing colon cancer. More recently oligosaccharides have also been shown to enhance calcium bioavailability in humans and animal studies have shown that prebiotic oligosaccharides can improve bone calcium concentration and structure.

9.4 References

1. Diplock A, Aggett P, Ashwell M, Bornet F, Fern E, Roberfroid M. Scientific Consensus of Functional Foods in Europe: Consensus document. *British Journal of Nutrition* 1999; 81: 1–27
2. Salminen S, Bouley C, Boutron-Ruault M-C, Cummings J, Franck A, Gibson G, Isolauri E, Moreau M-C, Roberfroid M, Rowland I. Functional Food Science and Gastrointestinal Physiology and Function. *British Journal of Nutrition* 1998; 80: 147–171
3. Hosono, A. In *Functions of Fermented Milk: Challenges for Health Sciences.* Barking: Elsevier Science Publishers Ltd, 66–77, 1992
4. Mims C, In: *Medical Microbiology*. London: Mosby, 3.1–3.3, 1993
5. Berg RD. The indigenous gastrointestinal microflora. *Trends in Microbiology* 1996; 4: 430–435
6. Holzapfel WH, Haberer P, Snel J, Schillinger U, Huis in't Veld, J. Overview of gut flora and probiotics. *International Journal of Food Microbiology* 1998; 41: 85–101
7. Gronlund MM, Salminen S, Mykkanen H, Kero P, Lehtonen OP. Development of intestinal bacterial enzymes in infants – relationship to mode of delivery and type of feeding. APMIS 1999; 107: 655–660
8. Cummings JH. *The large intestine in nutrition and disease.* Danone Chair Monograph, Brussels: Institut Danone 1997
9. Gibson GR, Roberfroid MB. Dietary manipulation of the human colonic microbiota: introducing the concept of prebiotics. *Journal of Nutrition* 1995; 125: 1401–1412
10. Fuller R, Gibson GR. Modification of the intestinal microflora using probiotics and prebiotics. *Scandinavian Journal of Gastroenterology* 1997; 32: 28–31
11. Orrhage K, Lidbeck A, Rafter J. In: Hill MJ (ed) *Role of gut bacteria in Human Toxicology and Pharmacology*. London: Taylor & Francis, pp 263–282, 1995
12. Metchnikoff E. In: Prolongation of Life. London; William Heinemann, 1907
13. Tissier H. Traitment des infections intestinales par la methode de transformation de la flore bacterienne de l'intestine. *C.R. Soc. Biologie* 1906; 60: 359–361
14. *Lactobacillus casei* strain Shirota. Yakult Central Institute for Microbiological Research, Tokyo; Yakult Honsha Company Ltd, 1999
15. Goldin B, Gorbach S, Saxelin M, Barakat S, Gualteri L, Salminen S. Survival of Lactobacillus species (strain GG) in the human gastrointestinal tract. *Digestive Diseases and Sciences* 1992; 37: 121–138
16. O'Sullivan M, Thornton G, O'Sullivan G, Collins J. Probiotic bacteria: myth or reality? *Trends in Food Science and Technology* 1992; 3: 309–314
17. Fuller RJ. A review: Probiotics in man and animals. *Applied Bacteriology* 1989; 66: 365–378
18. Huis in't Veld J, Havenaar R. Probiotics in health in man and animals. *J. Chem. Tech. Biotech* 1991; 51: 562–567
19. Huis in't Veld J, Shortt C. In: Leeds A & Rowland I (eds) Gut Flora and Health – Past, Present and Future. *The Royal Society of Medicine International Consortium and Symposium Series 6*, pp 27–36, 1996
20. Ouwehand AC, Kirjavainen PV, Shortt C, Salminen S. Probiotics: mechanisms and established effects. 1999 *International Dairy Journal*; 9: 43–52
21. Marteau P, Minekus M, Havenaar R, Huis in't Veld. Survival of lactic acid bacteria in a dynamic model of the stomach and small intestine: validation and effect of bile. *Journal of Dairy Science* 1997; 80: 1031–1037
22. Kullen JM, Amann MM, O'Shaughnessy MJ, O'Sullivan DJ, Busta FF, Brady LJ. Differentiation of ingested and endogenous bifidobacteria by DNA fingerprinting demonstrates

the survival of an unmodified strain in the gastrointestinal tract of humans. *Journal of Nutrition* 1997; 127: 89–94
23. Spanhaak S, Havenaar R, Schaafsma G. The effect of consumption of milk fermented by *Lactobacillus casei* Shirota on the intestinal microflora and immune parameters in humans. *European Journal of Clinical Nutrition* 1998; 52: 899–907
24. Wolf B, Garleb M, Ataya D, Casas I. Safety and tolerance of *Lactobacillus* reuterii in healthy adult male subjects. *Microbial Ecology in Health and Disease* 1995; 8: 41–50.
25. Dunne C, Murphy L, Flynn S, O'Mahoney L, O'Halloren S, Feeney M, Morrissey D, Thornton G, Fitzgerald G, Daly C, Kiely B, Quigley G, O'Sullivan, G, Shanahan F, Collins, J. Probiotics: from myth to reality. Demonstration of functionality in animal models of disease and in human clinical trials *Antoine van Leeuwenhoek* 1999; 76: 279–292
26. Brassart D, Schiffrin EJ. The use of probiotics to reinforce mucosal defence mechanisms. *Trends in Food Science and Technology* 1997; 8: 321–326
27. Yuki N, Koichi W, Mike A, Tagami Y, Tanaka R, Ohwaki M, Morotomi M. Survival of a probiotic, *Lactobacillus casei* strain Shirota, in the gastrointestinal tract: Selective isolation from faeces and identification using monoclonal antibodies. *International Journal of Food Microbiology* 1999; 48: 51–57
28. Saxelin M, Ahokas M, Salminen S. Dose response on the faecal colonization of Lactobacillus strain GG administrated in two different formulations. *Microbial Ecology in Health and Disease* 1993; 6: 119–122
29. Salminen S, Isolauri E, Salminen E. Clinical uses of probiotics for stabilizing the gut mucosal barrier: successful strains and future challenges. *Antoine van Leeuwenhook.* 1996; 70: 347–358
30. Hamilton-Miller JMT. Probiotic remedies are not what they seem. *British Medical Journal* 1996; 312: 55–56
31. Hamilton-Miller JMT, Shah S, Winkler JT. Public health issues arising from microbiological and labelling quality of foods and supplements containing probiotic microorganisms. *Public Health Nutrition* 1998; 2: 2–8
32. Bio yoghurts on test. In: *Health Which*, pp 92–95, June 1997
33. Hamilton-Miller JMT, Gibson G. Nutrition discussion forum – efficacy studies of probiotics: a call for guidelines. *British Journal of Nutrition* 1999; 82: 73–75
34. Adams MR, Marteau P. On the safety of lactic acid bacteria from food. *International Journal of Food Microbiology* 1995; 27: 263–264
35. Donohue D, Salminen S, Marteau P. Safety of probiotic bacteria. In: Salminen S, von Wright A (eds). *Lactic acid bacteria: microbiology and functional aspects.* New York: Marcel Dekker Inc, pp 369–384, 1998
36. Salminen S, von Wright A, Morelli L et al. Demonstration of safety of probiotics – a review. *International Journal of Food Microbiology* 1998; 44: 96–106
37. Fonden R, Mogensen G, Tanaka R, Salminen S. Culture containing diary products: effects on intestinal microflora, human nutrition and health – current knowledge and future perspectives. IDF Bulletin 2000: 352
38. Demonstration of safety of probiotics – a review. *International Journal of Food Microbiology* 1998; 44: 96–106
39. Saxelin M, Chuang NH, Chassy B, Rautelin H, Mäkelä PH, Salminen S, Gorbach SL. Lactobacilli and bacteremia in Southern Finland. 1989–1992. *Clinical Infectious Diseases* 1996; 22: 564–566
40. Saxelin M, Rautelin H, Salminen S, Mäkelä P. The safety of commercial products with viable *Lactobacillus* strains. *Infectious Diseases in Clinical Practice* 1996; 5: 331–335
41. Michetti P, Dorta G, Wiesel P, Brassart D, Verdu E, Herranz M, Felley C, Porta N, Rouvet M, Blum A, Corthesy-Theulax I. Effect of whey-based culture supernatant of lactobacillus acidophilus (johnsonii) La1 on Helicobacter pylori infection in humans. *Digestion.* 1999; 60: 203–209
42. Guandalini S, Pensabene L, Abu Zikri M, Amil Dias J, Gobio Casali L, Hoekstra H, Kolacek S, Massar K, Micetic-Turk D, Papadopoulou A, Salazar de Sousa, J, Sandhu B, Szajewska H, Weizman Z. *Journal of Paediatric Gastroenterology and Nutrition.* 2000; 30: 54–60

43. Naidu AS, Bidlack WR, Clemens RA, Probiotic spectra of lactic acid bacteria *Critical reviews in Food Science and Nutrition.*1999; 38: 13–126
44. Shortt C. Host-Microflora interface in Health and Disease *Trends in Food Science and Technology* 1999; 10: 182–185
45. MacFarlane G, Cummings J. Prebiotics and probiotics: can regulating the activities of intestinal barrier benefit health? *British Medical Journal* 1999; 318: 999–1003
46. Roberfroid MB. Fructo-oligosaccharide malabsorption: benefit for gastrointestinal functions. *Curr Opinion Gastroenterology* 2000; 16: 173–177
47. Delzenne N, Roberfroid MB. Physiological effects of non digestible oligosaccharides. *Lebensm Wiss u Technol* 1994; 27: 1–6
48. Cummings JH, Roberfroid MB. A new look at dietary carbohydrate: chemistry, physiology and health. *Eur J Clin Nutr* 1996; 51: 417–423
49. Roberfroid M, Slavin J. Resistant carbohydrates. *Crit Rev Food Sci Nutr* 2000; 40(6): 461–480
50. Roberfroid MB, Delzenne N. Dietary Fructans. *Ann Rev Nutr* 1999; 18: 117–143
51. Roberfroid MB, Van Loo JAE, Gibson GR. The bifidogenic nature of chicory inulin and its hydrolysis products. *J Nutr* 1998; 128: 11–19
52. Masai T, Wada K, Hayakawa K. Effects of soybean oligosaccharides on human intestinal flora and metabolic activities. *Jpn J Bacteriol* 1987; 42: 313–329
53. Wada K, Watabe J, Mizutani J, Tomoda M, Suzuki H, Saitoh Y. Effects of soybean oligosaccharides in a beverage on human fecal flora and metabolites. *Nippon Nogeikagaku Kaishi* 1992; 68: 127–135
54. Tanaka R, Takayama H, Morotomi M, Kuroshima T, Uetama S, Matsumoto K, Kuroda A, Mutai M. Effects of administration of TOS and *Bifidobacterium breve* 4006 on the human fecal flora. *Bifidobacteria Microflora* 1983; 2: 17–24
55. Ito M, Deguchi Y, Miyamori A, Kikuchi H, Matsumoto K, Kobayashi Y, Yajima T, Kan T. Effect of administration of galacto-oligosaccharides on the human fecal microflora, stool weight and abdominal sensation. *Microbial Ecology Health Dis.* 1990; 3: 285–292
56. Ito M, Kimura M, Deguchi Y, Miyamori-Watabe A, Yajima T, Kan T. Effects of transgalactosylated disaccharides on the human intestinal flora and their metabolism. *J Nutr Sci Vitaminol* 1993; 39: 279–288
57. Yoneyama M, Mandai T, Aga H, Fujii K, Sakai S, Katayama Y. Effects of 4^G-*b*-D-Galactosylsucrose (Lactosucre) intake on intestinal flora in healthy men. *Nippon Eijo Skokuryo Gakkaishi* (*J Jpn Soc Nutr Food Sci*) 1992; 45: 101–107
58. Kohmoto T, Fukui F, Takatu H, Machida Y, Arai M, Mitsuoka T. Effect of isomaltooligosaccharides on human fecal flora. *Bifidobacteria Microflora* 1988; 7: 61–69
59. Mizutani T. Properties and use of palatinose oligosaccharides. *New Food Industry* 1991; 33: 9–16
60. Imaizumi K, Nakatsu Y, Sato M, Sedarnawati Y, SuganoM. Effects of xylooligosaccharides on blood glucose, serum and liver lipids and cecum short-chain fatty acids in diabetic rats. *J Agric Biol Chem* 1991; 55: 199–205
61. Gibson GR, Rastall RA, Roberfroid MB. Prebiotics. In: Gibson GR & Roberfroid MB (eds) *Colonic Microbiot, Nutrition and Health,* 1st edn. Dordrecht: Kluwer Academic Publishers, pp 101–148, 1999
62. Franck A. Prebiotics in consumer products. In: Gibson GR & Roberfroid MB (eds) *Colonic Microbiot, Nutrition and Health,* Dordrecht: Kluwer Academic Publishers, pp 291–300, 1999
63. Van Loo J, Coussement P, De Leenheer L, Hoebregs H, Smits G. On the presence of inulin and oligofructose as natural ingredients in the western diet. *Crit Rev Food Sci Nutr* 1995; 35: 525–552
64. Moshfegh AJ, Friday JE, Goldman JP, Chug Ahuja JK. Presence of inulin and oligofructose in the diets of Americans. *J Nutr* 1999; 129: 1407–1411
65. Pudjono G, Barwald G, Amanu S. Activity of inulinase of certain strains of *Bifidobacterium* and their effects on the consumption of foods containing inulin and other fructans. In: Fuchs A (ed) *Inulin and inulin containing crops,* Amsterdam: Elsevier, pp 373–379, 1993

66. Dumortier V, Brassart C, Bouquelet S. Purification and properties of a β-galactosidase from *Bifidobacterium bifidum* exhibiting a transgalactosylation reaction. *Biotechnol Appl Biochem* 1994; 19: 341–354
67. Bach Knudsen KE, Hessov I. Recovery of inulin from Jerusalem artichoke (*Helianthus tuberosus* L.) in the small intestine of man. *Br J Nutr* 1995; 74: 101–113
68. Ellegärd L, Andersson H, Bosaeus I. Inulin and oligofructose do not influence the absorption of cholesterol or the excretion of cholesterol, Ca, Mg, Zn, Fe or bile acids but increase energy excretion in ileostomy subjects. *Eur J Clin Nutr* 1997; 51: 1–5
69. Molis Ch, Flourie B, Ouarne F, Gailing MF, Lartigue S, Guibert A, Bornet F, Galmiche JP. Digestion, excretion and energy value of fructooligosaccharides in healthy humans. *J Am Clin Nutr* 1996; 64: 324–328
70. Andersson HB, Ellegärd LH, Bosaeus IG. Nondigestibility characteristics of inulin and oligofructose in humans. *J Nutr* 1999; 129: 1428–1430
71. Gibson GR. Dietary modulation of the human gut microflora using prebiotic inulin and oligofructose. *J Nutr* 1999; 129 (suppl): 1438–1441
72. Rao AV. Dose-response effects of inulin and oligofructose on intestinal bifidogenesis effects. *J Nutr* 1999; 129 (suppl): 1442–1445
73. Hunter JO, Truffnell Q, Lee AJ. Controlled trial of oligofructose on the management of irritable bowel syndrome. *J Nutr* 1999; 129: 1451–1453
74. Catala I, Butel MJ, Benssada M, Popot F, Tessedre AC, Rimbault A, Szilit O. Oligofructose contributes to the protective role of *Bifidobacteria* in experimental necrotising enterocolitis in quails. *J Med Microbiol* 1999; 48: 89–94
75. Roberfroid MB. Caloric value of inulin and oligofructose. *J Nutr* 1999; 129: 1436–1437
76. Delzenne N, Aertssens J, Verplaetse H, Roccaro M, Roberfroid M. Effect of fermentable fructo-oligosaccharides on mineral, nitrogen and energy digestive balance in the rats. *Life Sci* 1995; 57: 1579–1587
77. Ohta A, Ohtsuki M, Baba S, Adachi T, Sakat T, Sakaguchi E. Calcium and magnesium absorption form the colon and rectum are increased in rats fed fructooligosaccharides. *J Nutr* 1995; 125: 2417–2424
78. Scholz-Arhens KE, Schaafsma G, van den Heuvel EGH, Schrezenmeir J. Effects of prebiotics on mineral metabolism. *Am J Clin Nutr* 2001; 73: 459–464
79. Van den Heuvel EGHM, Muys T, van Dokkum W, Schaafsma G. Oligofructose stimulates calcium absorption in adolescents. *Am J Nutr* 1999; 69: 544–548
80. Coudray C, Bellange J, Castiglia-Delahaut C, Rémésy C, Vermorel M, Demigné C. Effect of soluble and partly soluble dietary fibres supplementation on absorption and balance of calcium, magnesium, iron and zinc in healthy young men. *Eur J Clin Nutr* 1997; 51: 375–380
81. Prosky L. Inulin and oligofructose are part of the dietary fibre complex. *J Assoc Off Analyt Chem Int* 1999; 82: 223–226
82. Hoebregs H. Fructans in foods and food products, ion-eschange chromatographic method: collaborative study. *J Assoc Off Analyt Chem Int* 1997; 80: 1029–1037
83. Reddy BS, Hamid R, Rao CV. Effect of dietary oligofructose and inulin on colonic preneoplastic aberrant crypt foci inhibition. *Carcinogenesis* 1997; 18: 1371–1374
84. Rowland IR, Rumney CJ, Coutts JT, Lievense LC. Effect of *Bifidobacterium longum* and inulin on gut bacterial metabolism and carcinogen-induced aberrant crypt foci in rats. *Carcinogenesis* 1998; 19: 281–285
85. Pierre F, Perrin P, Champ M, Bornet F, Meflah K, Menanteau J. Short-chain fructooligosaccharides reduce the occurrence of colon tumors and develop gut-associated lymphoid tissue in Min mice. *Cancer Res* 1997; 57: 225–228
86. Rumney C, Rowland I. Non-digestible oligosaccharides: potential anticancer agents? *BNF Nutr Bull* 1995; 20: 194–203
87. Roberfroid MB. Concepts in functional foods: the case of inulin and oligofructose. *J Nutr* 1999; 129 (suppl): 1398–1401
88. Delzenne NM, Kok NN. Biochemical basis of oligofructose-induced hypolipidemia in animal models. *J Nutr* 1999; 129 (suppl): 1467–1470

89. Trautwein EA, Rieckhoff D, Erbersdobler HF. Dietary inulin lowers plasma cholesterol and triacylglycerol and alters biliary bile acid profile in hamsters. *J Nutr* 1998; 128: 1937–1943
90. Jackson KG, Taylor GRJ, Clohessy AM, Williams CM. The effect of the daily intake of inulin on fasting lipid, insulin and glucose concentrations in middle-aged men and women. *Br J Nutr* 1999; 82: 23–30
91. Williams CM. Affects of inulin and oligofructose on lipid parameters in humans. *J Nutr* 1999; 129 (suppl): 1741–1473
92. Delzenne N. The hypolipidemic effect of inulin: when animal studies help to approach the human problem. *Br J Nutr* 1999; 82: 3–4
93. Van Loo J, Cummings J, Delzenne N, Englyst H, Franck A, Hopkins M, Kok N, MacFarlane G, Newton D, Quigley M, Roberfroid M, van Vliet T, van den Heuvel E. Functional food properties of non-digestible oligosaccharides: a consensus report from ENDO project (DGXII AIRII-CT94–1095). *Br J Nutr* 1999; 81: 121–132

10 Phytoestrogens and Health

Janet Cade, Victoria Burley, and Sara Kirk

10.1 Introduction

10.1.1 Phytoestrogens – What are They and Where do we Find Them?

Phytoestrogens are compounds that are naturally present in almost all plant foods to a varying degree. They include several different classes of chemical compounds known as isoflavones, coumestans and lignans (Fig. 1). These compounds are structurally similar to the human hormone oestradiol, which is the most potent form of oestrogen [1]. Oestrogen is known to be of key importance in the maintenance of female reproductive health and bone density and is also believed to have a cardioprotective effect in pre-menopausal women. For these reasons, phytoestrogens are being viewed as potentially important in the development and management of a range of human diseases, including heart disease and some forms of hormone-sensitive cancers.

Phytoestrogens are known to produce a broad spectrum of biological activity and according to the dose, are capable of both oestrogenic or anti-oestrogenic effects [2]. They bind to oestrogen receptors in many tissues, but are not able to stimulate a full oestrogenic response [3]. In other words they have a mild effect compared to the natural oestrogens produced by our own bodies.

Initial interest in phytoestrogens developed following observations of reduced fertility in animals fed diets containing rich sources of phytoestrogens, such as red clover [4]. Interest then switched to their activity in humans, when it was postulated that some of the phytoestrogens could also explain (at least in part) why diets containing large amounts of plant foods are associated with lower mortality and morbidity in adult life [5]. However, one of the main problems encountered in studying the effects of these compounds is the large number of different substances incorporated within the phytoestrogen group. For example, at least 15 different types of isoflavones have been identified in foods. It is therefore very difficult to isolate the particular components responsible for a certain biological effect. This may partly explain why much of the evidence surrounding the role of phytoestrogens is often unclear and even conflicting. Further research is therefore needed before any definitive conclusions can be drawn about the use of phytoestrogens in disease management. This chapter aims to provide a summary of the evidence, along with guidance on how phytoestrogens might be best incorporated into our diets.

10.1.2 Isoflavones

To date, the bulk of research on phytoestrogens has been conducted on the isoflavone class of phytoestrogens. It is these compounds which have been thought in particular to have a protective effect against disease.

There are three main families of isoflavones, called genistein, daidzein and glycitein. These are formed when the body converts the isoflavone forms by removing the glucose on the side chain to make the aglycone form (genistein, daidzein and glycitein) prior to absorption or further metabolism by the body. The extent to which any further metabolism occurs appears to vary considerably between individuals and is influenced by the rest of the diet. For example, when a high carbohydrate diet is consumed, this generates increased intestinal fermentation by bacteria in the gut, with more biotransformation of phytoestrogens occurring. During this process, daidzein is converted to equol, a compound that has an oestrogenic potency which is much higher than its precursor daidzein [6].

Although isoflavones are generally found in legumes, soya beans and soya bean products are a particularly rich source [7]. However, the type of isoflavone found in soya-based foods is dependent upon the method of processing used. For example, non-fermented soya foods, like Tofu, contain greater levels of glucosides, while fermented soya foods, like Tempeh, contain greater levels of aglycones. Second generation soya foods, such as tofu yoghurt contain much less isoflavone than the original soya bean due to processing losses. Soya milk can be produced either from the whole bean (which has a rather beany flavour) or from isolated soy protein. Both these products have similar levels of isoflavones. A serving of 500 ml of soya milk per day can provide isoflavone intakes similar to that consumed by Japanese and Chinese people consuming a traditional diet. These levels of intake (around 25–50 mg/day) have been shown to have a cholesterol lowering effect in some studies [8]. Soya milk consumption may therefore be one of the ways in which people might consider supplementing their diet with phytoestrogens to achieve this benefit.

10.1.3 Coumestans

A large number of coumestans have been isolated from plants but only a few have been shown to have oestrogenic properties. Although, the metabolism of coumestans has not yet been fully characterised [1] it is thought that coumestrol, found in soy protein, is one of the most oestrogenic phytoestrogens studied.

Although split peas and some other legumes contain small amounts of coumestrol, the richest sources of coumestans in foods are found in sprouted seeds such as clover and alphalpha.

10.1.4 Lignans

Lignans are widespread in plants as lignin, which confers rigidity to plant cell walls. Plant lignans exist as diglucosides which are converted by colonic bacterial flora to the mammalian lignans, the diphenols: enterodiol and enterolactone. These latter compounds are structurally similar to oestradiol. As lignins have such an important structural role in plants they are widely found in plant foods. They are also found in soya beans and other legumes, wholegrain breads, brown rice, peanuts and fresh fruit and vegetables [4]. Not surprisingly, plasma lignan levels have been reported to be up to 10 times higher in vegetarians compared to omnivores [9, 10], reflecting the higher intakes found in a vegetarian diet.

10.2 Dietary Intake

Because of the relative novelty of interest in the role of phytoestrogens and difficulties encountered with their isolation and analysis, there is a lack of information about the phytoestrogen content of many food items. This is particularly the case for processed foods that contain some soya products, where levels of phytoestrogens may be variable due to losses that occur through processing. Until recently, most work on determining the presence of phytoestrogens in food has used urine and blood levels of isoflavones and lignans as a marker for food intake. Urinary levels of lignans are greater than isoflavone levels in individuals consuming a western diet, indicating the more widespread availability of lignans in the diet. Far Eastern intakes of isoflavones are around 30 mg/day, compared to negligible amounts (less than 1 mg/day) in people consuming more Western diets. Intakes of 50 mg/day of isoflavones will have significant endocrine effects [11]. To put this into the context of pharmacological doses of oestrogens, 20 g of soya bean sprouts contains 70 ppm coumestrol, equivalent to a daily dose of 0.5 diethylstilboestrol equivalents whereas the "morning after" pill contains 50,000 equivalents (Notis).

Table 1 shows some of the major dietary sources of phytoestrogens in the diet.

Studies looking at dietary intake of phytoestrogens in an American population found the main source of isoflavones to be peas and beans, the main source of coumestans to be broccoli and the main source of lignans to be fruits (other than citrus fruit) [12].

Urinary and blood levels of isoflavones and lignans increase after consumption of a soya bean or linseed supplement. Blood levels can increase within 30 minutes of consumption and begin to decline after 5 hours post-ingestion, although elevated levels remain at 24 hours [4].

When soya is consumed regularly, plasma isoflavone levels are found to be much greater than normal plasma oestradiol levels. Dose and duration of intake are therefore major factors affecting the clinical and biological outcome of a phytoestrogen-rich diet.

Dietary supplements containing isoflavones are appearing on the market, as "natural" hormone replacement therapies. Some breads containing seeds are

Table 1. Phytoestrogen content of some common foods[1]

Food	Daidzein mg/100 g	Genistein mg/100 g	Coumestrol mg/100 g	Enterodiol µg/100 g	Enterolactone µg/100 g
Tofu	4.2	6.3			
Soya milk	0.5	0.4			
Miso	20.0	23.2			
Tempeh	11.3	16.4			
Soya sauce	0.8	0.5			
TVP	3.0	6.7			
Rapeseed (unprocessed)				155	975
Wheat bran				298	269
Brown rice				128	169
Pea (dried)			8.1		
Peas (frozen)				62	60
Lentils				119	278
Baked beans				96	269
Broccoli				65	161
Garlic				326	81
Carrot				62	284
Pear				69	112

Missing values do not imply that the food does not contain the phytoestrogen, rather that the values are not available.

[1] Main source of information NOTIS CD-ROM (Institute of Food Research, Norwich, UK).

being marketed as phytoestrogen-rich. Since the impact of these modified foods and supplements on health has yet to be fully established, it is not possible to form a clear opinion about their suitability for the general public.

10.2.1 Baby Foods

As more information becomes available about the effects of exposure to environmental endocrine modulators [13], there has been some recent concern that like oestrogens, the consumption of phytoestrogen-rich soya-based infant formulae might have adverse effects on sexual development and fertility. Although, there is no evidence that there are any ill effects of soya consumption on the fertility of populations that normally use large quantities of soya, animal studies show that a hormonal imbalance in early life may lead to reproductive problems [13]. Examination of the isoflavone concentration of infant formulae showed that cows' milk based samples were below the limit of detection, but soya-based samples had concentrations ranging from 18 mg-33 mg isoflavone per litre of made up formula. Therefore, a 1–2 month infant would potentially consume in

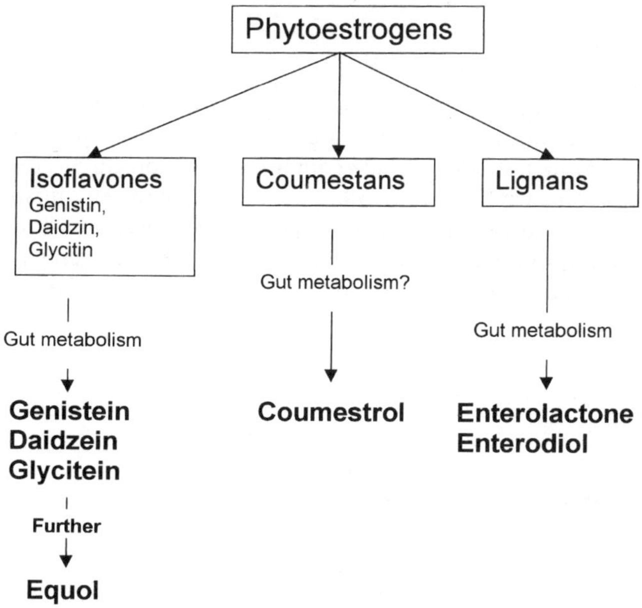

Fig. 1. Classification of phytoestrogens

the region of 5 mg isoflavone/kg body weight per day. Isoflavones circulate at concentrations that are 13,000–22,000-fold higher than plasma oestradiol concentrations in early life [14]. However, since the metabolism of isoflavones is still poorly understood it is not clear what the implications are of these findings. Levels of isoflavones in formulae have not increased over recent years and in general, breast milk (or cows' milk formulae) is the preferred source of nutrition for infants. As more suitable hydrolysate-based formulae become available the clinical grounds for recommending the use of soya-based formulae are reducing. Parents who have been advised by their doctor or other health professionals to use soya-based formulae are recommended to continue, as the benefits are thought to outweigh any potential risks. The Panel on Child and Maternal Nutrition of the Committee on Medical Aspects of Food and Nutrition Policy states that since it is possible that there may be adverse effects from phytoestrogens in soya products, including soya based formulae, the precautionary principle should be applied i.e unless there are definite clinical grounds for using soya based formulae other milks should be provided [15, 16].

10.2.2 Key Points

- Soya derived foods are the main dietary sources of isoflavonoids.
- Lignans are widely consumed in the diet.
- Far Eastern diets contain higher levels of phytoestrogens than Western diets.
- There is currently no evidence of harm from soya-based infant formulae.

10.2.3 Effects on Health

Heart disease, breast cancer, prostate cancer, osteoporosis and menopausal symptoms share a common epidemiology in that they are all rare in populations which consume traditional diets containing soya products compared with western populations, where soya products are consumed only in small quantities. Cross-sectional studies show higher phytoestrogen levels in urine and plasma in populations at lower risk of these diseases. Thus, it has been suggested that supplementing the diet with phytoestrogens may reduce the risk of developing these diseases.

10.3 Heart Disease

10.3.1 Phytoestrogens May Reduce Blood Cholesterol Levels

The main established risk factors for coronary heart disease (CHD) are raised serum cholesterol, raised blood pressure and smoking. Prior to their menopause, women are better protected than men from developing raised cholesterol levels by the production of oestrogen. This is one reason why men are more prone to heart disease than women. It also explains why post-menopausal women are at increased risk of heart disease, when oestrogen levels fall, leading to a rise in cholesterol levels.

Cholesterol reduction can be achieved by reduction in saturated fat intake in the diet or by drugs. Oestrogens in hormone replacement therapy and the anti-oestrogen drug Tamoxifen also lower LDL-cholesterol, the type of cholesterol associated with raised serum cholesterol levels [4]. A recent meta-analysis of 38 controlled clinical trials has concluded that consumption of soya protein rather than animal protein significantly decreases blood cholesterol, LDL cholesterol and triglycerides [17]. This review also suggested that phytoestrogens may account for around 60–70% of the effects seen. The American Food and Drug Administration has recently agreed that label claims can be made on certain food products to the effect that regular consumption of soya protein may help to reduce the risk of heart disease. The mechanism by which this occurs is not yet clear, although the beneficial effects are not seen in animals fed soya protein with the isoflavones removed [18]. However, the non-starch polysaccharide (NSP or dietary fibre) found in soya beans might also account for some of the cholesterol lowering effects found. Isolated isoflavone concentrates (which may be used in dietary supplements) have not been shown to have a positive effect on lowering cholesterol. This suggests that there may be some other component at work that enhances the hypocholesterolaemic effect of phytoestrogens [19, 20].

10.3.2 Other Possible Effects of Phytoestrogens on CHD Risk

Oestrogen has acute beneficial effects on vascular reactivity and longer-term effects on critical steps in the pathogenesis of atherosclerosis. Phytoestrogens appear to have potent beneficial effects on the arterial wall. The phytoestrogens have certain similarities to 'designer hormones' which are being developed to retain their beneficial effects on the cardiovascular system and the skeleton without having cancer promoting effects on the breast and endometrium [21]. Isoflavones have antioxidant properties and may contribute to reducing the oxidation of lipids [22]. This will protect against the first stages of atherosclerosis whereby oxidatively damaged LDL-lipoproteins form foam cells in the lining of the arteries.

One study has found that an important measure of arterial health, systemic arterial compliance, was significantly improved in perimenopausal and menopausal women taking soya isoflavones to about the same extent as may be achieved with conventional hormone replacement therapy [20].

Genistein, in particular, has been shown to have an effect on tyrosine kinases and may influence the cellular processes that lead to atherosclerosis. It has also been found to affect the clotting process in vitro, inhibiting platelet aggregation and acting as a thromboxane-receptor agonist. Some of these effects occur at low levels of intake [4]. Future research should assess the potential therapeutic effects of phytoestrogens in vivo.

10.3.3 Key Points

- Phytoestrogen foods *may* lower blood cholesterol.
- Isoflavones act as antioxidants.
- Genistein may affect the blood-clotting process.

10.4 Cancer

10.4.1 General Effects of Phytoestrogens

There is mounting evidence that phytoestrogens in the diet may reduce the risk of certain cancers. In vitro studies have suggested numerous mechanisms by which isoflavones may be cancer preventive. The weakly oestrogenic diphenols formed from phytoestrogens influence sex-hormone production, metabolism and biological activity, intracellular enzymes, protein synthesis, growth factor action, malignant cell proliferation, differentiation, cell adhesion and angiogenesis in such a way as to make them strong candidates for a role as natural cancer-protective compounds. Their effect on some of the most important steroid synthesising enzymes may result in beneficial changes in hormone concentrations and action in the cells, thereby inhibiting the development of cancer [23].

Phytoestrogens bind to the oestrogen-receptors without stimulating a full oestrogenic response. They antagonise oestradiol and can act as both oestrogens and anti-oestrogens. In animal models, soya bean products generally reduce tumours induced by chemical carcinogens. This effect has been attributed to the anti-oestrogenic characteristics of isoflavones [4]. Lignans and isoflavonoids may affect uptake and metabolism of sex hormones by participating in the regulation of plasma serum hormone binding globulin levels. In this way, they may inhibit cancer cell growth, like some flavonoids, by competing with oestradiol for the type II oestrogen binding sites [24]. In vitro, genistein can inhibit the growth of a wide range of hormone dependent and independent cancer cells and can inhibit the metastatic activity of both breast and prostate cancer cells [3]. These effects tend to occur at levels higher than can be easily achieved by dietary intake in free-living populations. On the other hand, some phytoestrogens have been shown to have proliferative (i.e. cancer promoting) effects through oestrogen receptor mediated pathways at rather lower concentrations [1].

Independent of the actions of phytoestrogens themselves is the fact that diets higher in plant products are usually rich in antioxidants and other micronutrients and lower in fat, which may result in leaner individuals with less potential for the synthesis of oestradiol in adipose tissue. Further research is needed to determine the relative health benefits of other dietary components compared with phytoestrogens.

10.4.2 Breast Cancer

There is evidence to suggest that the consumption of phytoestrogens is inversely related to breast cancer risk, although their effects seem to be influenced by the dosage consumed, the presence of obesity and menopausal status. It has been hypothesised that obesity increases the risk of postmenopausal breast cancer in women consuming small quantities of phytoestrogens, but may not increase risk in women consuming larger quantities. This may occur by diminishing the binding capacity of stronger endogenous oestrogens to receptors. Such an association might partly explain the low breast cancer rates observed among postmenopausal Hispanic women despite their greater adiposity, an important risk factor for breast cancer. If this association could be demonstrated it would have important implications for reducing breast cancer risk through diet, using naturally occurring substances, particularly in women for whom postmenopausal obesity is an important health concern [25].

There is no direct evidence of reduced risk of breast cancer or recurrence of the disease from intervention studies using either phytoestrogen rich diets or supplements. However, phytoestrogen-rich diets and supplements are known to modulate menstrual cycle duration, which is indirectly related to breast cancer risk.

Pre-menopausal women who consumed a supplement containing 45 mg isoflavones per day showed a 2.5 day increase in the follicular phase of their menstrual cycle and reduced levels of follicle stimulating hormone and luteinizing hormone [11]. However, not all studies have shown this effect, and it may be dependent on the amount of phytoestrogens consumed. Nevertheless, longer cycles, which are typical of Asian women, have been associated with reduced risk of breast cancer. Furthermore, a meta-analysis of 9 studies (8 case-control and 1 cohort) showed some evidence of a small reduction in pre-menopausal breast cancer risk associated with soya consumption. However, the number of studies was small and the measurement of soya intake was crude. Interpretation of these studies was complicated by the generally low consumption of soya products in the studies on non-Asian populations, and the fact that similar reductions in risk were associated with widely varying soya intakes. The relationship is confused further by the results of some studies that have indicated potentially adverse effects of soya on breast cancer risk. On balance, it is therefore too early to recommend that women increase their soya intake until further trials have been conducted [26].

10.4.3 Prostate Cancer

Prostate cancer is the most common hormone dependent cancer in men, with a rapidly rising incidence rate in the UK. The incidence rate of clinical prostate cancer in the USA among white men is 10–15 fold higher than the Japanese rate. However, the overall latent prostate cancer rate is only about 50% higher in the USA. (Latent prostate cancer being cancer which does not progress during life and is determined at postmortem or following surgical resection of the prostate.) This suggests that in some populations the growth of prostate tumours is slower or the onset occurs later in life. Although clearly, many lifestyle features may differentiate between these populations it has been speculated that the intake of soya bean foods may be a contributory factor.

There are no reports of clinical trials in which phytoestrogens have been demonstrated to reduce the incidence rates of prostate cancer [27]. However, one small trial of feeding soya to men with prostate cancer found that the men given a fermented soya drink had a slower rise in the production of prostate specific antigen (a marker of prostate cancer) compared to the placebo group over 6 months [28]. Furthermore, isoflavone levels in prostatic fluid are much higher in Hong Kong and Chinese men consuming soya than Portuguese and British men [29]. Tofu consumption has been associated with reduced risk of prostate cancer in Japanese men (although the difference did not quite reach statistical significance) [30].

At present there is no evidence that phytoestrogens are either beneficial or detrimental to men who are undergoing treatment for prostate cancer.

10.4.4 Other Cancers

The evidence from case-control studies in which soya bean intake has been assessed has been reviewed by Messina et al. [31]. In general, they concluded that high intakes of soya appear to protect against lung and stomach cancer. Studies conducted on rats, however, have indicated that raw soya products may cause pancreatic carcinomas. Carcinoma levels are reduced on cooking and processing soya flour, and there is no epidemiological evidence that human populations consuming soya bean are at greater risk of pancreatic cancer [32].

10.4.5 Key Points

- Epidemiological evidence and in vitro studies suggest a protective role for phytoestrogens in a number of cancers.
- There is no direct evidence from clinical trials to support this as yet.
- For people with existing hormone-dependent cancers, supplementing the diet with phytoestrogens will probably not be harmful.

10.5 Osteoporosis

Osteoporosis is particularly prevalent in women during and after the menopause due to the loss of oestrogen that accelerates bone loss. Hormone-replacement therapy and Tamoxifen are known to slow down this bone loss. A synthetic phytoestrogen, Ipriflavone can inhibit bone-resorption in post-menopausal women, though its action is not thought to be due to association with oestrogen receptors [4]. Animal studies have shown that phytoestrogens, particularly coumestrol, can prevent bone loss by increasing bone formation at a rate which exceeds bone resorption [33].

It is likely that postmenopausal women may benefit from dietary supplementation with phytoestrogens to maintain bone mass. A recent trial in which a soya bean protein supplement (containing a relatively high dose of isoflavones) was consumed over 6 months demonstrated a clear improvement in bone mineral density in a group of postmenopausal women [34].

Epidemiological data on this issue is scarce and does not always support a protective effect. For example, in a 10-year follow up study among postmenopausal women in the Netherlands urinary isoflavone excretion was measured and compared with the rate of bone loss. Excretion of isoflavonoids did not differ between groups according to the rate of bone loss, although in multivariate analysis equol excretion was weakly positively associated with rate of bone loss in the five years after the menopause. Enterolactone excretion was significantly higher in the group with a high rate of bone loss. This positive association remained in multivariate analysis after adjustment for age, years since menopause, body mass index and intake of calcium, vegetable protein and dietary fibre. Enterolactone excretion is therefore likely to be an indicator of consumption of grains and legumes, however, it is not clear whether the observed positive association with rate of bone loss is a causal one. These results do not support a preventive effect of low, unsupplemented dietary intake of phytoestrogens on postmenopausal cortical bone loss. However, no conclusions can be drawn about effects of higher doses of phytoestrogens [34].

Soya intake has also been suggested to protect against bone loss by mechanisms that are independent of its oestrogenic effects. Soya foods are a good source of calcium and a high soya protein diet may prevent the urinary calcium loss seen with a high animal protein diet [1]. This may help to offset lower calcium intakes among vegetarians and vegans [3].

Osteoporosis has been predicted to be a new burden to public health in Asia. Currently, the incidence of osteoporosis-related fractures in Asia is lower than in most western communities. By the year 2050, however, 50% of the 6.3 million hip fractures that occur world wide will occur in Asians due to a combination of factors, including; an ageing population, a decrease in physical activity and westernization of lifestyles. The cost of treatment and cure for these patients will be large. Public health education is needed to encourage the Asian population to maintain their traditionally healthy lifestyle thereby reducing the risk factors for osteoporosis [36].

10.6 Key points

- A high phytoestrogen diet may protect against osteoporosis.
- There is not enough evidence to make clear recommendations on this issue.

10.7 Menopausal Symptoms

Although the menopause is an inevitable life event for women there is considerable variation across populations in the degree to which individuals suffer from side effects associated with falling oestrogen levels. In the developed world, it has been estimated that approximately 70% of women will suffer from some symptoms, typically hot flushes and sweats [6].

Oestrogen is known to modulate serotonergic function [37]. It has been suggested that oestrogen and serotonin are involved in reproductive-endocrine-related mood disorders: premenstrual syndrome and perimenopausal depression [38]. Low serotonin activity premenstrually has been associated with depression and effects on appetite [39]. Oestradiol replacement therapy showed a significant increase in urinary 5-hydroxyindole acetic acid (5-HIAA) in post menopausal women due to enhanced serotonin turnover [40]. Since phytoestrogens exert weak oestrogenic effects, they may affect serotonin levels thereby playing a role in mood changes and cognitive function during the menopause.

Although there is considerable interest in the use of phytoestrogens as an alternative to classical HRT therapy [41], there is currently only limited hard evidence that the consumption of different phytoestrogens will have a significant impact on symptoms experienced. Until recently, much of the evidence on phytoestrogens has been provided by anecdotal reports or poorly conducted studies in which the results were complicated by a large placebo effect.

One study of Japanese women found that estimated isoflavone intake from total and fermented soya products was lower in women who experienced hot flushes compared to those without [42]. A randomised double-blind controlled trial of soya flour or wheat flour supplements, in 58 postmenopausal women with menopausal symptoms found a significant reduction in hot flushes in the soya group compared to the wheat group over 12 weeks [43]. In another study 97 post-menopausal women were randomized to a diet containing soya foods or their normal diet [41]. Only a small oestrogenic effect on vaginal cytology was found after 4 weeks on the soya diet. A third trial also found that a phytoestrogen-rich diet over 12 weeks alleviated hot flushes and vaginal dryness symptoms [44]. However, two recent trials did not find any conclusive improvement in menopausal symptoms [45, 46] and it is clear that there is a need to look in more detail at the potential effects and mechanisms of phytoestrogens on the oestrogenisation of post-menopausal women.

10.7.1 Key Points

- Although research on the effects of phytoestrogens on menopausal symptoms is in its infancy, the evidence suggests that there may be some benefits, particularly in reducing hot flushes.
- This area is worthy of further investigation.

10.8 Potential Adverse Effects

Since phytoestrogens act as weak oestrogens it is possible that adverse effects associated with oestrogens, such as deep vein thrombosis, may also be a potential risk with consumption of phytoestrogen supplements or phytoestrogen-rich foods [47].

There has been increasing concern about the effect of oestrogen-like compounds on the reproductive health of males, both human and animal. In theory, phytoestrogens and structurally related compounds could harm the reproductive health of males by acting as antioestrogens. Exposure to diethylstilbestrol (DES) (a synthetic oestrogen) induces changes in the developing reproductive tract of males. It is possible that oestrogen-like substances other than DES alter sexual differentiation in males and account for the increasing incidence of developmental disorders of the reproductive tract in men and wild animals. Phytoestrogens (coumestans, isoflavonoids, flavonoids, and lignans) present in numerous edible plants are quantitatively the most important environmental oestrogens when their hormonal potency is assessed in vitro. Oestrogenic effects in wildlife have been described but the evidence for the role of phytoestrogens is indirect and only seen under conditions of excessive exposure. Animal studies have shown that in doses comparable to the daily intake from soya-based feed, isoflavonoids such as genistein were oestrogen – agonists in the prostate of adult laboratory rodents. In neonatal animals, no persistent effects were observed. In contrast, the rat appears to be sensitive to phytoestrogens during development in terms of male sexual behaviour and development. The changes were similar but not identical to those seen after neonatal treatment with DES, although higher doses of phytoestrogens were needed [48].

10.9 Conclusions and Recommendations

Despite considerable research activity in the field of phytoestrogens, conclusive evidence is lacking for most of the postulated health benefits of these compounds.

Phytoestrogens are generally found in soya-based foods, fruit, vegetables, legumes and whole grains. Recommendations for healthy eating suggest that we consume at least five portions of fruit and vegetables per day [49]. Encouraging people to eat a diet rich in fruit and vegetables and whole grain cereals will automatically increase the phytoestrogen content of the diet and may have a whole range of positive consequences for health.

Until further results from clinical trials are available it is still too soon to recommend consumption of phytoestrogen-rich dietary supplements. However, if people choose to consume these products there is little evidence that they will do any harm.

10.10 References

1. Kurzer MS, Xu X. Dietary phytoestrogens. Annual Review of Nutrition 1997; 17: 353–381
2. Setchell KD, Borriello SP, Hulme P, Kirk DN, Axelson M. Nonsteroidal estrogens of dietary origin: possible roles in hormone- dependent disease. American Journal of Clinical Nutrition 1984; 40: 569–578
3. Anderson JJB, Anthony M, Messina M, Garner SC. Effects of phyto-oestrogens on tissues. Nutrition Research Reviews 1999; 12: 75–116
4. Bingham SA, Atkinson C, Liggins J, Bluck L, Coward A. Phyto-oestrogens: where are we now? British Journal of Nutrition 1998; 79: 393–406
5. Thorogood M, Mann J, Appleby P, McPherson K. Risk of death from cancer and ischaemic heart disease in meat and non- meat eaters BMJ 1994; 308: 1667–1670
6. Setchell KD, Cassidy A. Dietary isoflavones: biological effects and relevance to human health. Journal of Nutrition 1999; 129: 758S–767S
7. Reinli K, Block G. Phytoestrogen content of foods–a compendium of literature values. Nutrition & Cancer 1996; 26: 123–148
8. Crouse JR, III, Morgan T, Terry JG, Ellis J, Vitolins M, Burke GL. A randomized trial comparing the effect of casein with that of soy protein containing varying amounts of isoflavones on plasma concentrations of lipids and lipoproteins. Archives of Internal Medicine 1999; 159: 2070–2076
9. Adlercreutz H, Fotsis T, Lampe J et al. Quantitative determination of lignans and isoflavonoids in plasma of omnivorous and vegetarian women by isotope dilution gas chromatography-mass spectrometry. Scandinavian Journal of Clinical Laboratory Investigations 1993; 215: 5–18
10. Adlercreutz H, Fotsis T, Watanabe S et al. Determination of lignans and isoflavonoids in plasma by isotope dilution gas chromatography-mass spectrometry. Cancer Detection and Prevention 1994; 18: 259–271
11. Cassidy A, Bingham S, Setchell K. Biological effects of isoflavones in young women: importance of the chemical composition of soyabean products. British Journal of Nutrition 1995; 74: 587–601
12. de Kleijn MJJ, van der Schouw YT, Wilson PWF, Grobbee DE, Jacques PF. Intake of dietary phytoestrogens in postmenopausal women. The Framingham Heart Study. Third International Symposium on the role of soy in preventing and treating chronic disease 1999. Washington, USA. 1999

13. Golden RJ, Noller KL, Titus-Ernstoff L et al. Environmental endocrine modulators and human health: an assessment of the biological evidence. Critical Reviews in Toxicology 1998; 28: 109–227
14. Setchell KD, Zimmer-Nechemias L, Cai J, Heubi JE. Isoflavone content of infant formulas and the metabolic fate of these phytoestrogens in early life. [86 refs]. American Journal of Clinical Nutrition 1998; 68: 1453S–1461S
15. MAFF Joint Food Safety and Standards Group. Plant oestrogens in soya-based infant formulae. Food Surveillance Information Sheet No. 167. 1998
16. National Dairy Council. Advice about soya-based infant formulae. Issue 1, 1999/2000. 1999. National Dairy Council Nutrition Service. 1999
17. Anderson JW, Johnstone BM, Cook-Newell ME. Meta-analysis of the effects of soy protein intake on serum lipids. New England Journal of Medicine 1995; 333: 276–282
18. Anthony MS, Clarkson TB, Hughes CLJ, Morgan TM, Burke GL. Soybean isoflavones improve cardiovascular risk factors without affecting the reproductive system of peripubertal rhesus monkeys. Journal of Nutrition 1996; 126: 43–50
19. Greaves KA, Zhang L, Williams K, Parks J, and Wagner JD. Phytoestrogen and intact soy protein administrations differ in their effects on plasma lipids and lipoproteins. Symposium on Phytoestrogen Research Methods, Tuscon, Arizona. 1997
20. Nestel PJ, Yamashita T, Sasahara T et al. Soy isoflavones improve systemic arterial compliance but not plasma lipids in menopausal and perimenopausal women. Arteriosclerosis Thrombosis & Vascular Biology 1997; 17: 3392–3398
21. St Clair RW. Estrogens and atherosclerosis: phytoestrogens and selective estrogen receptor modulators. Current Opinion In Lipidology 1998; 9: 457–463
22. Kapiotis S, Hermann M, Held I, Seelos C, Ehringer H, Gmeiner BM. Genistein, the dietary-derived angiogenesis inhibitor, prevents LDL oxidation and protects endothelial cells from damage by atherogenic LDL. Arteriosclerosis, Thrombosis & Vascular Biology 1997; 17: 2868–2874
23. Adlercreutz H, Mazur W. Phyto-oestrogens and Western diseases. Annals of Medicine 1997; 29: 95–120
24. Adlercreutz H, Mousavi Y, Clark J et al. Dietary phytoestrogens and cancer: in vitro and in vivo studies. Journal of Steroid Biochemistry and Molecular Biology 1992; 41: 331–337
25. Horn-Ross PL. Phytoestrogens, body composition, and breast cancer. Cancer Causes & Control 1995; 6: 567–573
26. Trock B, White Butler L, Clarke R, and Hilakivi-Clarke L. Meta-analysis of soy intake and breast cancer. Third International Symposium on the role of soy in preventing and treating chronic disease. Washington, DC, USA. 1999
27. Mydlo JH, Kanter JL, Kral JG, MacChia RJ. The role of obesity and diet in urological carcinogenesis. British Journal of Urology International 1999; 84: 225–234
28. Barken I, Eliaz I, Baranov IE, and Geller J. The effect of two soy preparations on prostate-specific antigen levels in patients with prostate cancer and the correlation of prostate-specific antigen changes with plasma genistein. Third International Symposium on the role of soy in preventing and treating chronic disease. 1999. Washington, DC, USA
29. Morton MS, Matos-Ferreira A, Abranches-Monteiro L et al. Measurement and metabolism of isoflavonoids and lignans in the human male. Cancer Letters 1997; 114: 145–151
30. Severson RK, Nomura AM, Grove JS, Stemmermann GN. A prospective study of demographics, diet, and prostate cancer among men of Japanese ancestry in Hawaii. Cancer Research 1989; 49: 1857–1860
31. Messina MJ, Persky V, Setchell KD, Barnes S. Soy intake and cancer risk: a review of the in vitro and in vivo data. Nutrition & Cancer 1994; 21: 113–131
32. Bingham SA, Setchell KD, Cassidy A. Soya and safety. New Scientist 1994; 46–47
33. Arjmandi BH, Alekel L, Hollis BW et al. Dietary soybean protein prevents bone loss in an ovariectomized rat model of osteoporosis. Journal of Nutrition 1996; 126: 161–167
34. Potter SM, Baum JA, Teng H, Stillman RJ, Shay NF, Erdman JW Jr. Soy protein and isoflavones: their effects on blood lipids and bone density in postmenopausal women. American Journal of Clinical Nutrition 1998; 68: 1375S–1379S

35. Kardinaal AF, Morton MS, Bruggemann-Rotgans IE, van Beresteijn EC. Phyto-oestrogen excretion and rate of bone loss in postmenopausal women. European Journal of Clinical Nutrition 1998; 52: 850–855
36. Kao PC, P'eng FK. How to reduce the risk factors of osteoporosis in Asia. Chung Hua i Hsueh Tsa Chih - Chinese Medical Journal 1995; 55: 209–213
37. Joffe H, Cohen LS. Estrogen, serotonin, and mood disturbance: where is the therapeutic bridge? Biological Psychiatry 1998; 44: 798–811
38. Rubinow DR, Schmidt PJ, Roca CA. Estrogen-serotonin interactions: implications for affective regulation. Biological Psychiatry 1998; 44: 839–850
39. Dye L, Blundell JE. Menstrual cycle and appetite control: implications for weight regulation. Human Reproduction 1997; 12: 1142–1151
40. Lippert TH, Filshie M, Muck AO, Seeger H, Zwirner M. Serotonin metabolite excretion after postmenopausal estradiol therapy. Maturitas 1996; 24: 37–41
41. Baird DD, Umbach DM, Lansdell L et al. Dietary intervention study to assess estrogenicity of dietary soy among postmenopausal women. Journal of Clinical Endocrinology & Metabolism 1995; 80: 1685–1690
42. Nagata C, Shimizu H, Takami R, Hayashi M, Takeda N, Yasudat K. Hot flushes and other menopausal symptoms in relation to soy product intake in Japanese women. Climacteric 1999; 2: 6–12
43. Murkies AL, Lombard C, Strauss BJG, Wilcox G, Burger HG, Morton MS. Dietary flour supplementation decreases post-menopausal hot flushes: Effect of soy and wheat. Maturitas 1995; 21: 189–195
44. Brzezinski A, Adlercreutz H, Shaoul R, Shmueli A, Reosler A, Schenker JG. Short-term effects of phytoestrogen-rich diet on postmenopausal women. Menopause 1997; 4: 89–94
45. Albertazzi P, Pansini F, Bottazzi M, Bonaccorsi G, De Aloysio D, Morton MS. Dietary soy supplementation and phytoestrogen levels. Obstetrics & Gynecology 1999; 94: 229–231
46. Gamache PH, Acworth IN. Analysis of phytoestrogens and polyphenols in plasma, tissue, and urine using HPLC with coulometric array detection. Proceedings of the Society for Experimental Biology & Medicine 1998; 217: 274–280
47. Wiseman H. Dietary phytoestrogens: disease prevention versus potential hazards. Nutrition and Food Science 1997; 1: 32–38
48. Santti R, Makela S, Strauss L, Korkman J, Kostian ML. Phytoestrogens: potential endocrine disruptors in males. Toxicology & Industrial Health 1998; 14: 223–237
49. World Health Organisation. Diet, nutrition and the prevention of chronic disease. 1990. Geneva, WHO. Technical Report Series no. 797

11 Dietary Supplements and their Role in the Prevention and Treatment of Coronary Heart Disease

Peter Jackson, Lawrence Ramsay, and Erica Wallis

11.1 Introduction

Despite all the strategies to prevent coronary heart disease (CHD) and the advances in the treatment of existing disease it remains one of the major causes of morbidity and mortality in the Western world. The lifetime risk of coronary events is such that most adult men will suffer a coronary event and the proportion of women similarly affected, although smaller, is still sizeable. Prevention of CHD is one of the UK Government's key targets set out in 'Saving lives: our healthier nation' and whilst rates of CHD have begun to fall, the UK remains one of the world's black spots for coronary disease [1]. Although much public concern is about death from HIV and cancer, heart disease remains numerically a much greater threat to health. Even in the developing world CHD, once infrequent compared with deaths due to infectious diseases, is now an important disease.

The pathological process behind coronary heart disease is the accumulation of cholesterol rich lipid material in plaques beneath the inner surface of arterial walls. Fatty streaks in the artery walls start at an early age and the plaques progressively increase in size. Eventually some reach a size where they bulge into the vessel lumen and markedly impede the flow of blood. When this type of obstruction occurs in a critical artery, such as that supplying blood to the muscle of the heart, it becomes impossible for flow to increase in response to the extra demand when physical activity or emotion increases the work of the heart. The lack of oxygenated blood to the heart muscle causes the typical pain of angina. Whilst most atheromatous plaques are covered by smooth endothelium, in others this breaks down exposing the blood to the fatty material inside the plaque which triggers off the formation of a blood clot. The artery is then completely blocked by the clot filling the lumen already diminished by plaque. The blood supply to the muscle beyond the blockage is completely cut off leading to muscle death. This is the mechanism underlying a myocardial infarction (MI) or heart attack. Diet has a key role in the aetiology of coronary heart disease. Only a moderate proportion of circulating cholesterol comes from dietary sources although there is a very high correlation between the amount of saturated fat eaten and total concentration of cholesterol in the blood. The seven-countries study [2] showed a very strong link between the mean consumption of saturated fat and the development of coronary heart disease in the following 10 years for 16 closely defined cohorts. Those populations where saturated fat intake was high also had high rates of coronary disease. Earlier less rigorous studies based on national food balance sheets or household surveys rather than actual consumption showed negative correlations between the prevalence of CHD and the amounts of vegetable and flour produced or imported.

Even accepting that diet has a major role in the aetiology of vascular disease it may be questioned why effort should be expended in discovering the role of individual dietary supplements rather than that of drugs or changes in diet itself. Drugs are often perceived by patients as foreign chemicals unlike the natural connotations of food and there remains a resistance to the taking of drugs however large the benefit. Although the national diet is slowly changing towards a model perceived as healthy progress in this direction is painfully slow. In a population study [3] looking at the willingness of patients to take treatment to prevent coronary heart disease, 16% of those approached were unwilling to take long term drug therapy despite this offering a reduction of one third in CHD events or mortality without major adverse effects. Dietary supplements are seen as natural, and if shown to be of benefit, would have the dual advantages of avoiding both foreign chemicals and the personal effort required for a major change in long established dietary habits. In counties including the UK where healthcare is paid for by the government, food supplements also have the advantage of being paid for by individuals rather than by the government who pick up the major proportion of the bill for any new drug treatment.

11.2 Evidence

Before considering studies about individual food components it is important to consider the types of evidence necessary to deduce benefit and safety. Much of the evidence used to promote food supplements is based on biological plausibility or on the results of cross-sectional epidemiological or prospective cohort studies. This contrasts with the emphasis on the randomised controlled trial or even meta-analyses of such trials as the basis for the use of drugs for the treatment and prevention of disease. Some of this difference in approach may be due to the vast resources of the pharmaceutical industry based on high profits sustainable from the sale of monopoly products. Randomised controlled trials of the type needed to investigate food components are extremely expensive costing many tens of millions of pounds. Different criteria are used by a doctor deciding whether to prescribe a drug and a member of the public choosing whether to purchase a food supplement. Government regulations for food additives and supplements are quite different from those for drugs. For the latter the Medicines Control Agency requires evidence of both safety and efficacy. In nearly every case they will demand evidence of efficacy based on the results of randomised placebo controlled trials. Even when considering safety the requirements differ when considering drugs and food supplements or additives.

Randomised controlled clinical trials do have serious limitations particularly due to the exclusion of many subjects to whom their results will subsequently be applied [4]. However they are not subject to the huge range of biases inherent in cross-sectional epidemiological and prospective cohort studies [5]. A further limitation of this type of epidemiological approach to determine the likely benefit of an individual food component is that food is a complex biological matrix containing a multitude of components. There is often a high correlation between the nutrient or food component being investigated and other nutrients in the diet. This makes it difficult to assess the impact of single food components on health status. Thus it is difficult to change dietary intake of β-carotene and folate independently as both nutrients are found in a number of commonly eaten foods. The exception to this limitation is the rare occurrence when a high proportion of the population studied already take supplements of one particular component.

Biological plausibility alone should never be the basis for a change in dietary policy. We can not be certain that all the possible pathways bearing upon a particular problem are fully understood. It is embarrassing to recall the effects of early diets for patients with diabetes which were based on our limited understanding of the disease [6]. In these diets carbohydrates were replaced by fat resulting in a massive increase in total blood cholesterol concentration in a population already at high risk of vascular disease due to low concentrations of the protective high density lipoprotein (HDL) cholesterol. In the past less stringent standards were required before recommending changes in lifestyle following the somewhat cynical argument that whilst such changes were unlikely to be of major benefit they were also unlikely to be the source of major harm. This overlooks not only the possibility of direct harm, especially when individual food component are used at higher than normal dose, but also the financial and psychological cost to the individual consequent upon a change in lifestyle. There is also the possibility that in following such change members of the public might neglect seeking medical advice which, for some people, might be to take drug treatment capable of achieving a much greater benefit.

11.3 Early Attempts at Dietary Modification to Prevent CHD

The initial emphasis on dietary modification to prevent CHD was placed on taking constituents out of the diet [7], particularly saturated fats. This approach was not found to be uniformly effective and whilst some individual studies [8] showed a reduction in sudden death due to CHD, benefit from this type of dietary change was not universal [9]. The explanation for this may be found in the poor response of total cholesterol in the blood to restriction of saturated fat and cholesterol in the diet of free living subjects. Short term metabolic ward studies [10] of diets with reduced total fat intake, restricted cholesterol, and an increase in the ratio of polyunsaturated to saturated fat showed a dramatic response in total blood cholesterol concentration. This was not seen when the same diets were used in larger longer term studies in free living individuals [11]. It is not known whether this discrepancy in the effect of low fat diets is due to any response being transient or to the difficulty experienced by many participants in adhering to the diet when alternative sources of food were freely available. Many commentators have invoked poor compliance as the most likely explanation, suggesting that increased efforts in patient education might overcome the problem. However huge resources, far greater than might be available in routine practice, were used in the Multiple Risk Factor Intervention Trial [12] (MRFIT) and yet the response in blood cholesterol concentration remained small. Enthusiasts for such diets overlook the fact that poor compliance is as much a comment on the long term palatability of the diet as it is on the commitment of the trial participants. The other issue often raised when considering the practical implications of these findings is that of responders and non-responders. Many doctors and dieticians claim to have patients who achieve substantial falls in blood cholesterol concentrations in response to a low saturated fat diet. They suggest that a trial of diet is worthwhile as responders would benefit and may avoid the need for drug treatment. However if some subjects benefit from large falls in total cholesterol and yet the mean response for all advised to take the diet is close to zero then logically other patients must respond to the diet with an increase in total cholesterol and be at greater risk of CHD. No thought has been given as to how any harm caused to these subjects might be reversed.

11.4 The Diet Trials

A rational approach to dietary change to prevent CHD in countries where the risk is high would be to introduce diets similar to those taken in countries where the incidence of CHD is low. One such diet studied is called the 'Mediterranean diet' as it is based on the diet consumed by the Cretan people living around the western Mediterranean.

In the Lyon Diet Heart Study [13] patients less than 70 years of age of either sex, recovering from a myocardial infarction within the previous 6 months were allocated either to standard hospital dietetic advice or to advice and assistance to follow a Mediterranean style diet including more bread, more root and green vegetables, more fish, less meat, fruit taken every day and butter replaced by margarine. The study was stopped early following an interim analysis as both cardiac and overall mortality were found to be 70% lower in the group of patients receiving the Mediterranean style diet. A study with a similar dietary modification [14] was reported for Indian men who were recovering from a recent myocardial infarction. In this study one group was advised to take the standard Step 1 diet of the American Heart Association. This low fat diet is a low cholesterol, reduced saturated fat diet. The comparator group received the same advice to follow the Step 1 diet but in addition were advised to increase their intake of fruit, vegetables, nuts and grain products. After three years subjects receiving the additional advice, especially those who had lost weight, had benefited with lower rates of non-fatal myocardial infarction and overall mortality. Both these diet studies can be criticised as control and intervention groups received differing amounts of support and attention during follow-up, mainly to avoid them comparing notes. However it is of note that neither of the control groups adhered to the dietary advice given at the outset, as well as the intervention group. Also increased supervision provides non-specific support which has been shown in other studies to be beneficial in patients post MI.

Furthermore, in the Lyon study differences between groups were not limited to the dietary advice. Patients in the intervention group were provided with free supplies of a special rapeseed oil based margarine to replace the butter and cream normally part of their diet. This margarine had a similar fatty acid composition to olive oil but was slightly more rich in linoleic acid and α-linolenic acid. Thus the intervention tested was not simply that of adhering to a Mediterranean diet. Nevertheless the findings of these two similar studies would support the concept that some dietary modification produces benefit in subjects with pre-existing CHD.

11.4.1 Fish

A number of studies have looked at the association between fish consumption and the prevalence of coronary heart disease. We performed a structured overview [15] of these studies in 1998 and found an inconsistency amongst the prospective epidemiological studies. The control group in the MRFIT, the Western Electric [16] and Zutphen [17] studies all showed a significant inverse relationship between the consumption of oily fish and the subsequent risk of death from CHD. A similar but non-significant trend was evident in the 14 year follow-up data for Swedish men and women [18] and a case control study [19] of Italian men came to the same conclusion. However studies similar in size and duration of follow-up have failed to show any protective effect of fish consumption. The Health Professional follow-up study, the 4 year follow-up data from the Physicians Health Study [20], 14 year prospective data for Norwegian men and 12 year follow-up data for Japanese men in Honolulu [21] all failed to show any association. These apparently contradictory findings can best be explained by methodological flaws in some studies with lack of adjustment for other cardiovascular risk factors. In addition whilst the estimates of fish consumption were based on that at the time of initial screening, many of the men increased fish consumption during follow-up. This would weaken any observed link between fish consumption and difference in the rates of subsequent CHD. Finally it is possible that there is a threshold relationship in which a protective effect of oily fish consumption is only seen in populations whose usual diet contains little oily fish.

In the absence of clear consistent evidence from the epidemiological studies we are dependent upon the results of intervention studies for our conclusions about the role of oily fish in preventing CHD. No primary prevention studies of increased consumption of oily fish or fish oil supplements in people free of vascular disease have been published. Of the studies in secondary prevention only the Diet and Reinfarction Trial (DART) [22] is truly satisfactory, the others are far too small or methodologically flawed. In this trial men who had already suffered a myocardial infarction were allocated either to a control group or intervention groups receiving advice to increase fibre, reduce fat or increase consumption of oily fish in a factorial design. Thus some were advised to increase fibre alone, some to reduce fat and a third group to eat more oily fish whilst other groups received advice about two foodstuffs in combination and one group received advice about all three dietary modifications. The men in the groups randomised to receive advice about increasing their intake of oily fish consumed an average of 43 g more oily fish per day than those groups not receiving this advice. After two years they had a 29% lower all cause mortality mainly due to a reduction in CHD deaths.

All the studies considered so far have investigated oily fish consumption as part of the diet rather than as fish oil supplements. Eating fish as part of a meal could have a beneficial effect simply by replacing other more harmful food sources. Until recently we had relatively little information about the effect of the addition of fish oil as a supplement. The investigators of the DART study [22] did provide information about the results in a subgroup of men who were unable to tolerate the oily fish and were therefore given fish oil capsules. Whilst the findings are consistent with those of the principal analysis for all subjects the men receiving the fish oil capsules were not randomised into this category but received the capsules only because of their inability to eat sufficient oily fish. This analysis must therefore be interpreted with caution. Recently however the Italian GISSI[1] prevention trial has reported its investigation of the use of fish oil supplements [23]. This again was another factorial design study in men recovering from a myocardial infarction. The other intervention in this study was that of supplementing the diet with vitamin E. Rather than being encouraged to eat oily fish, men in the fish oil study limbs were supplied with capsules containing an average of 865 mg n-3 polyunsaturated fatty acids (PUFA) to take daily. Men receiving these capsules benefited after 3.5 years by a 10% reduction in the primary endpoint of death, non-fatal myocardial infarction or non-fatal stroke. Of particular note was that this benefit, although smaller than expected, was achieved on a background of modern drug treatment for the prevention of recurrent CHD.

11.4.2
Nuts

The Indian post-MI trial [24] demonstrated benefit from a diet which included a switch to consumption of nut oil both as whole nuts and through the use of ground nut oil. Superficially nuts might be thought an unlikely nutrient to help prevent vascular disease. Their fat content is high and in animal studies peanuts have been seen as atherogenic [25]. However a large cohort study of Adventists [26] suggested that cardiac mortality was much lower in those subjects who ate more than 5 helpings of nuts per week. In this study Californian Adventist families were contacted in the 1970 s and asked to complete a validated food frequency questionnaire. People who participated were contacted each year afterwards to detect new cases of CHD. This population is particularly convenient as religious strictures on smoking and alcohol consumption limit heterogeneity and the possibility of bias due to confounding of nut intake with other risk factors. Those participants who ate nuts more than 4 times each week experienced 48% fewer fatal CHD events and 51% fewer non-fatal MIs during follow-up.

[1] Gruppo Italiano per lo Studio della Sopravvivenza nell'Infarto miocardico.

Table 1. Intervention trials of fish oil supplements or advice to eat more oily fish – effect on cardiovascular mortality and non-fatal MI

Study	Relative risk	Confidence interval
DART	0.65	0.48–0.87
GISSI	0.83	0.70–0.97
Overall	0.78	0.68–0.90

Data from the massive US Nurses Health study [27], a prospective observational study, also points to a protective effect conferred by nut consumption. In this study of women's health, food questionnaires were sent out in 1980, 1984, 1986 and 1990 to women on a register of qualified nurses. Participants were then contacted every two years to detect new cases of coronary heart disease. Deaths were detected either by family reporting or via the National Death Index. Compared with women who almost never ate nuts, those who had nuts once each week had a 26% lower risk of developing CHD and in those who ate nuts 2–4 times each week the risk was 44% lower. Unfortunately nut consumption correlated with less smoking, a better family history of premature ischaemic heart disease, more hormone replacement therapy (HRT) use, greater vigorous exercise and a higher dietary intake of polyunsaturated fat. It is only after 'correction' for these possible confounding factors that the true effect of nut consumption could possibly be tested. There remains the concern that there are possible unrecognised confounders not taken into account or even that the correction is not robust.

Whilst nuts do contain a high proportion of fats much of this is polyunsaturated with a lower content of saturated fat. Certain nuts such as walnuts have a particularly high content of the polyunsaturated fatty acid α-linolenic acid and a short term experimental study [28] showed that a diet supplemented by 84 g of walnuts per day produced a favourable change in the lipid profile with a fall in low density lipoprotein (LDL) and, despite a small fall in HDL cholesterol, a significant reduction in the LDL:HDL ratio. The lipid content of other nuts is slightly less attractive and as noted above nuts such as peanuts have been seen as atherogenic. However in the Nurses Health study the trend for lower ischaemic heart disease persisted, albeit attenuated, when the analysis was limited to peanut consumption.

11.4.3 Fibre

Dietary fibre intake has also been shown to be inversely related to the risk of developing coronary heart disease in the prospectively investigated US health professionals cohort [29]. This relationship persisted even when corrected for non-dietary risk factors for vascular disease, dietary saturated fat, vitamin E, total energy intake and alcohol consumption. The dietary source of fibre most strongly linked to reduced risk of MI was that derived from cereal as opposed to fibre from vegetable and fruit sources. The gradient of the association would suggest that a 10 g increase in cereal fibre per day relates to a decrease in the risk of subsequent myocardial infarction by as much as 19%.

One of the limbs of the DART study [22] rarely mentioned is that investigating the effect of advice to increase dietary fibre. Whilst men given advice to increase their intake of oily fish did gain some benefit those advised to increase their intake of dietary fibre showed no reduction in the rate of recurrence of vascular events. If anything subjects taking larger amounts of fibre had a small but non-significant increase in the rate of further events.

11.5 Homocysteine

Classical homocystinuria is a rare inherited disease caused by homozygous deficiency of cystathionine β-synthase a key enzyme for homocysteine degradation [30]. These patients have very high blood concentrations of homocysteine and suffer from a number of defects including dislocation of the lens of the eye, intellectual handicap and skeletal deformities. In addition they have a high risk of vascular disease such that by the age of 30 the majority have sustained an arterial vascular event. In the 1970s it was grasped that homocysteine concentrations much lower than those seen in classical homocystinuria but still above average might be associated with premature vascular disease. In 1976 Wilcken [31] studied patients undergoing angiography for the investigation of possible CHD and found that patients with demonstrable disease were much more likely to have a high level of homocysteine in response to an oral methionine load when compared with subjects with normal coronary arteries or healthy controls. Subsequently several cross-sectional epidemiological studies have shown a negative correlation between plasma homocysteine concentrations and coronary heart disease. The interpretation of these studies is made difficult as blood homocysteine concentrations tend to rise after any vascular event. Prospective studies have been much less consistent. Perhaps longer studies investigating patients at very high risk of CHD have been more likely to show a positive relationship between blood homocysteine concentrations and the development of vascular disease. Any epidemiological study is however complicated because the blood concentration of homocysteine is also highly correlated with other strong risk factors for vascular disease such as high blood pressure and diabetes. Thus any deficiency in the measurement of the traditional risk factor such as a variable assay, a limited range of values, or deficiencies in the statistical model such as non-linearity might falsely suggest a causal role for homocysteine. Further indirect evidence for a role of homocysteine in the development of vascular disease comes from studies investigating the association between the risk of vascular disease and a common polymorphism of the enzyme methylenetetrahydrofolate reductase (MTHFR) and between vitamin B_6 intake and heart disease. The enzyme MTHFR is key in the remethylation of homocysteine to methionine in tissues outside the liver and vitamin B_6 is an essential cofactor in this pathway. There is a common polymorphism of the enzyme MTHFR for which 10–13% of white populations are heterozygotes and in them the concentration of homocysteine is moderately elevated. An early study [32] suggested that heterozygotes for this polymorphism were at increased risk of vascular disease although it has proved difficult to replicate this finding in all subsequent studies [33]. Vitamin B_6 was also investigated as one of the nutritional factors in the US Nurses Health study [34]. Those with the highest quintile of vitamin B_6 intake were 30% less likely to report a subsequent coronary event when compared with women in the lowest quintile.

The population importance of homocysteine is that high concentrations are seen in subjects with low intakes of folic acid and vitamins B_6 and B_{12}. If homocysteine truly is a powerful risk factor for vascular disease its inverse link with these nutrients might explain the protective effect of diets with large amounts of fruit and vegetables.

With the inconsistencies of the epidemiological data we are again having to await the outcome of the many intervention studies looking at the effect of folate or vitamin B_6 supplements on the risk of vascular disease. Blood concentrations of homocysteine fall in response to supplements of vitamins B_6, B_{12} or folic acid. In a meta-analysis [35] of the 12 short term randomised controlled trials of folic acid it was shown that a range of doses (0.5 mg – 5 mg per day) produced a 25% fall in the blood concentration of homocysteine. The fall was if anything greater in those with the highest concentrations of homocysteine or lowest folate intakes at baseline. Addition of vitamin B_{12} but not vitamin B_6 was associated with a small but statistically significant further decline. There are some data [36] to suggest that in patients with classical homocystinuria supplementation with folic acid and vitamins B_{12} and B_6 does reduce the incidence of cardiovascular disease. In the wider population the effects of relative folate deficiency may already be addressed to a limited degree by the progressive increase in the level of supplementation of foodstuffs with folate. The motivation for this is to prevent neural tube defects rather than avoiding vascular disease. Further investigation of the role of homocysteine is however of value as the dose of folate required to suppress homocysteine is probably much higher than that required to reduce the risk of neural tube defects. Folate supplementation is not without some possible risk and the increase in supplements to prevent neural tube defect has been strenuously resisted in the past. The concern is that patients with borderline vitamin B_{12} deficiency receiving folate supplements may go on to suffer the neurological sequelae of vitamin B_{12} deficiency, with subacute combined degeneration of the spinal cord, whilst the more easily recognised haematological presentation with anaemia is masked by the folate.

11.6 Antioxidants

In 1989 Steinberg [37] proposed the hypothesis that oxidised LDL had a pivotal role in the pathogenesis of atherosclerosis. This form of LDL but not native LDL is actively scavenged by macrophages which then transform into foam cells, the precursor to atheromatous lesions in arterial walls. Oxidised LDL is also a strong attractant to macrophages and is able to stimulate the release of growth factors which may contribute to its role in the development of atherosclerotic lesions.

There is considerable indirect evidence that oxidation of LDL may be important in promoting atherosclerosis. It is now known that the oxidation of LDL takes place in vivo [38]. In animal models of atherosclerosis caused by hypercholesterolaemia antioxidant drugs prevent the oxidation of LDL and delay the development of atheromatous lesions. There are a number of naturally occurring antioxidants in food especially β-carotene and vitamins C and E. It is therefore important to ascertain whether these should be used either to increase the supply in those with small amounts in their normal diet or used in supraphysiological doses to reduce the risk of CHD in people with a normal dietary intake.

11.6.1 Vitamin C

The most important antioxidant in terms of amount in the normal diet is vitamin C. A number of studies have looked at the association between vitamin C intake and the risk of developing CHD. Unfortunately these show inconsistent results. A large prospective epidemiological study in Finnish men and women [39] suggested that a high intake of vitamin C was associated with a reduced risk of death from CHD in women but not men. Similarly in separate observational studies in American men and women high intakes of vitamin C appeared to benefit only women [40,41]. A third American cohort study suggested that cardiovascular mortality was reduced in both sexes by vitamin C [42]. In the UK a cohort of subjects [43] free of vascular disease were invited by the Department of Health and Social Security in 1973 and 1974 to complete a 7 day food diary and the 20 year follow-up data for these people are now available. Even following adjustment for other known risk factors for vascular disease the risk of stroke in those with the highest intake of vitamin C was only half that of subjects with the lowest intake. Concentrations of ascorbic acid in the blood had a similar predictive value. Interestingly there was no suggestion of a lower rate of CHD in those with high vitamin C intakes.

Intervention studies with vitamin C have been even less encouraging although they are limited in number, small, and of short duration. The common endpoint reported for all studies was of overall mortality and a recent meta-analysis by Ness and colleagues [44] showed no evidence of benefit.

11.6.2 β-carotene

This antioxidant is abundant in fruit and vegetables and any protective effect might explain the apparent negative correlation between diets rich in these foods and the incidence of CHD. Jha and colleagues [45] recently reviewed the observational data relating to β-carotene and coronary disease. Taking all six observational studies together, there appeared to be a significant relative risk reduction when those with the highest intake or plasma concentration of β-carotene were compared with those with a low intake or plasma concentration. However individual observational studies comparing either subjects with low or high β-carotene intake have not consistently shown a protective effect. In two large Finnish studies only male smokers benefited by a 60% reduction in coronary events.

The results of the intervention studies of β-carotene have been uniformly disappointing. The primary aim of many of these studies was to investigate the effect of β-carotene supplements on protection against malignant disease. Therefore subjects with known risk factors for cancer, smokers and those exposed to asbestos, were included. Nevertheless data about the cardiovascular outcomes were also collected. These showed either no benefit or even a small detrimental effect of β-carotene supplementation. Davey-Smith and colleagues have performed a meta-analysis [46] of all these intervention studies which showed a small but statistically significant increase in the risk of cardiovascular death in participants who received β-carotene supplements.

11.6.3 Vitamin E

If anything vitamin E has been investigated more thoroughly than any other nutrient and the results of the observational studies show a consistent benefit in a reduction in vascular disease. Four very large prospective studies [47–50] with prolonged follow-up have been reported all of subjects free of vascular disease at the outset. Of note is that the two largest studies, including an analysis of US Nurses Health study showed only benefit in those subjects who used vitamin E supplements and only after these had been taken for more than two years. When subjects taking vitamin E supplements were excluded from these analyses there was no gradient of risk with intake. Thus if vitamin E is effective in protecting against coronary disease it needs to be taken in supraphysiological doses.

A number of interventional studies with vitamin E have been performed whilst others are ongoing or are about to be reported. The results so far are conflicting. Some [51–53], including the α-Tocopherol, β-Carotene Cancer Prevention Study (ATBC) used low doses and as might be predicted from the results of the observational studies, produced no significant effect on CHD of either benefit or harm. In contrast the Cambridge Heart Antioxidant Study (CHAOS) study [54] reported a 68% reduction in non-fatal MI in East Anglian men with radiologically confirmed coronary heart disease in response to vita-

Table 2. Intervention trials of β-carotene supplements – effect on cardiovascular mortality

Study	Relative risk	Confidence interval
Finnish male smokers	1.11	1.01–1.23
Smokers & asbestos workers	1.20	0.98–1.45
Skin cancer patients	1.09	0.93–1.27
US doctors	1.15	0.80–1.65
Overall	1.13	1.04–1.23

min E supplements of either 400 IU or 800 IU per day. However both total and cardiovascular mortality were increased but this was neither analysed nor mentioned in the paper. This trial was also criticised because of the change in the dose of vitamin E used part way through the study, the imbalance of the groups, the incomplete follow-up. In the GISSI prevention [23] study Italian men who had recently suffered a heart attack supplements of vitamin E were studied along with added n-3 PUFA in a factorial design. Thus one group received vitamin E alone, one PUFA alone, one both supplements and one neither. As discussed above the groups receiving fish oil gained some benefit. Men randomised to receive vitamin E at a dose of 300 mg per day gained no significant benefit. If anything in this study there was a trend towards a reduction in CHD mortality rather than non-fatal MI in contrast to the findings in the CHAOS study. The most recent controlled clinical trial investigating supplements of vitamin E to complete is the Heart Outcomes Prevention Evaluation study [55] (HOPE) which was also of a factorial design. In this trial the ACE inhibitor ramipril and vitamin E supplements at a dose of 400 IU per day were compared with placebo in men at high risk of CHD events due either to a history of previous CHD, stroke or peripheral vascular disease or diabetes plus one other risk factor such as high blood pressure, adverse cholesterol profile, smoking or microalbuminuria. The study reported no significant benefit in those men who received vitamin E supplements. Indeed if anything there was a fractional increase in the primary endpoint of MI, stroke, or cardiovascular death.

The reason for this discrepancy between observational studies and intervention studies is unclear. It might be because of the doses of supplement used or due to the inclusion of subjects who already had established vascular disease. Alternatively it might suggest that the observational studies results are due mainly to confounding.

It is tempting to suggest that as the antioxidant vitamins studied are part of our natural diet there is little to be lost by encouraging people to take supplements on the basis of the epidemiological studies alone. However the only strong evidence of a beneficial effect on CHD from these is for high doses of vitamin E. As Steinberg, the original proponent of the oxidised LDL hypothesis, points out

Table 3. Intervention trials of vitamin E supplements – effect on cardiovascular mortality and non-fatal MI

Study	Relative risk	Confidence interval
ATBC[a] primary	0.97	0.86 – 1.11
ATBC angina	1.01	0.72 – 1.42
ATBC previous MI	0.92	0.67 – 1.28
CHAOS	0.58	0.39 – 0.87
GISSI	1.01	0.89 – 1.14
HOPE	1.06	0.95 – 1.19
Overall	1.00	0.94 – 1.07

[a] α-Tocopherol, β-Carotene Cancer Prevention Study (ATBC).

[56] the safety of high doses of such antioxidant supplements in the long term is unproven. Indeed there are some preliminary data to suggest that high doses of vitamin E may increase the risk of haemorrahgic stroke.

11.7 Alcohol

One food to which there would be little resistance if it were advised as a supplement to avoid CHD is alcohol. Early cross-sectional studies showed a relationship between alcohol consumption and total mortality which was not monotonic [57]. Risk of vascular disease, particularly stroke, was certainly increased in people with a high alcohol consumption but there was also a slight excess of risk in those who were teetotal when compared with subjects who drank small amounts of alcohol. This apparent protective effect was initially thought due to an effect of wine consumption and would have been compatible with the oxidised LDL hypothesis as red wine is rich in antioxidant flavanoids. However subsequent analyses have confirmed lower risk associated with the consumption of small amounts of alcohol independent of the type of alcoholic beverage taken [58]. The mechanisms behind any possible benefit of alcohol are unclear. Certainly there is an association between alcohol consumption and increased concentrations of HDL cholesterol. There may also be a beneficial effect on clotting factors. Larger amounts of alcohol have certainly been associated with harmful effects on vascular health. Even moderate drinking is associated with an elevation in blood pressure and experimental studies show that this rise occurs soon after drinking contrary to previous expectations. There is also an independent association between binge drinking and stroke. The benefit of drinking wine was thought to explain the lower incidence of CHD in France compared with the UK despite the similarity of other CHD risk factors. This 'French paradox' has more recently been explained [59] by a much lower intake of saturated fat intake in France until recent years which, along with the long incubation time for vascular disease, might explain the observed difference in the rates of CHD. However the only data suggesting a benefit from alcohol consumption are those from observational studies and these almost universally from the investigation of older people. The evidence for benefit in early and middle adult life is minimal. Even if alcohol in low doses does protect against vascular disease this benefit will have to be carefully weighed against the clear increase in morbidity and mortality from cancers, cirrhosis and accidents with increasing consumption.

11.8 Plant Sterols and Stanols

One of the food industries most recent products aimed at improving health is cholesterol lowering margarine. Such products are based on plant derived sterols and work by blocking the absorption of dietary cholesterol from the gastrointestinal tract. As the sterols and stanols themselves are largely unabsorbed they are assumed to have a low potential for toxicity. There can be little doubt that such products are effective in lowering the cholesterol concentration in the blood. Short term studies [60] in volunteers demonstrated that 1.8 g or 2.6 g of sitostanol per day caused a 10.2% fall in total cholesterol over 12 months. This was associated with no serious adverse effects and was well tolerated by the volunteers in the study. However concerns have been voiced about possible phyto-oestrogenic activity of plant sterols and whether their immune modulating activity could be of any clinical significance. Safety is of paramount importance when such products could be taken by a significant proportion of the population over a very long period of time. Furthermore if the antioxidant vitamins do have any role in cardioprotection the benefit from reduced cholesterol produced by these food products must be weighed against any possible adverse effect secondary to reduced absorption of vitamins A, E and β-carotene. Being food supplements or additives the toxicity testing of plant sterols and stanols is quite different from that required of new drugs and being available for general sale there is no need to convince a sceptical medical profession. Earlier drug treatments shown to reduce cholesterol were associated with a significant increase in non-coronary morbidity and mortality which outweighed any benefit from reduced coronary disease. The more recently introduced HMG Co-A reductase inhibitors were only widely adopted in the UK when randomised controlled trials demonstrated a beneficial effect on overall mortality.

11.9 Conclusion

The overall picture of research into nutritional factors and their role in protecting against CHD is overwhelmingly one of highly suggestive observational studies followed by interventional studies which show no or even harmful effects. This has led some, perhaps because they are convinced by the indirect evidence, to question the utility of randomised controlled trials to answer questions relating to food supplements. Observational studies are, even when performed rigorously and incorporating all known safeguards, still open to confounding with some as yet unknown powerful risk factor. Randomised controlled trials in contrast are far less prone to bias and are unlikely, especially if repeatedly positive, to generate false positive results. Their problem is that they are performed in a tightly defined group of people quite different from those who might eventually select to take a food supplement. The question here is whether it is safe to extrapolate to groups other than those included in the trials. The duration of intervention studies might be considered too short to demonstrate the beneficial effects of supplements seen in much longer prospective observational studies. Certainly most clinical trials only investigate the effects of treatments over periods of 4–8 years whilst the development of atherosclerotic lesions takes many years. However the beneficial effects of a number of drugs or nutrients such as $n-3$ PUFAs have been confirmed by randomised controlled trials of this duration. It is of course possible that patients need to be exposed to some protective mechanisms for longer to receive benefit. Certainly the benefits of vitamin E seen in epidemiological studies were limited to subjects taking supplements for 2 years or longer with the greatest benefit been seen with very long exposures. The other difference between the observational and interventional studies has been the tendency to investigate people free of disease in the observational studies but those who already had established disease in the intervention studies. Once the disease is established the ability of food supplements to reverse the process could be limited. However this would contrast with the findings when new drugs are investigated that patients with established disease benefit to a much greater extent than those free of disease. This is because they are at greater risk of recurrence before treatment.

Using similar standards for evidence of benefit as those used for new drugs disappointingly few food supplements can be wholeheartedly endorsed as definitely reducing the risk of coronary heart disease. Clearly a change in diet from a standard Western diet to one with a reduced amount of saturated fat and a much greater proportion of fruit vegetables and nuts has an effect on the recurrence of further vascular events. However the individual components of such diets responsible for this benefit have yet to be isolated. Further progress is likely to be slow because the work involved in testing each individual factor is immense and costly. Any profits from the sale of food supplements is likely to be less than that from a drug of comparable effect because the lack of a patent makes exclusivity difficult and future profits smaller. Thus it is unlikely that the food industry alone will fund the necessary interventional research and governmental agencies have other priorities. It might be argued from the public health viewpoint that more could be gained by concentrating resources on educating the general population about the benefits of moving towards an overall 'healthy diet'. This avoids the need to ensure the safety of dietary components used at supraphysiological doses.

11.10 References

1. Great Britain. Dept. of Health, *Saving lives: our healthier nation*, presented to Parliament by the Secretary of State for Health by command of Her Majesty, July 1999
2. Keys A. *Seven countries*. Cambridge, Mass:, Harvard University Press, 1980
3. Nicholson K, Ramsay LE, Haq IU, Wallis EJ, Gharamani P, Jackson PR, Yeo WW. Factors affecting the acceptance of drug therapy to prevent myocardial infarction. *Br J clin Pharmac* 1999; 47: 580P
4. Chalmers I. Unbiased, relevant, and reliable assessments in health care. *BMJ* 1998; 317: 1167–1168
5. Feinstein AR. Epidemiologic analyses of causation: the unlearned scientific lessons of randomized trials. *Journal of Clinical Epidemiology*. 1989; 42: 481–489
6. Kaufmann RL, Assal JPh, Soeldner JS, Wilmshurst EG, Lemaire JR, Gleason RE. White P. Plasma lipid levels in diabetic children. Effect of diet restricted in cholesterol and saturated fats. *Diabetes*. 1975; 24: 672–679
7. Corr LA, Oliver MF. The low fat/low cholesterol diet is ineffective *European Heart Journal*. 1997; 18: 18–22
8. Hjermann I. Smoking and diet intervention in healthy coronary high risk men. Methods and 5 year follow-up of risk factors in a randomized trial. The Oslo study. Journal of Oslo City Hospital 1980; 30: 3–17
9. Ravnskov U. Cholesterol lowering trials in coronary heart disease: frequency of citation and outcome. *BMJ* 1992; 305: 15–19

10. Clarke R. Frost C. Collins R. Appleby P. Peto R. Dietary lipids and blood cholesterol: quantitative meta-analysis of metabolic ward studies. *BMJ*. 1997; 314: 112–117
11. Ramsay LE, Yeo WW, Jackson PR. Dietary reduction of serum cholesterol concentration: time to think again. *BMJ* 1991; 303: 953–957
12. Multiple Risk Factor Intervention Trial Research Group. Multiple risk factor intervention trial. Risk factor changes and mortality results. *JAMA* 1982; 248: 1465–1477
13. Mediterranean α-linolenic acid-rich diet in secondary prevention of coronary heart disease. De Lorgeril M, Renaud S, Mamelle N et. al. *Lancet* 1994; 343: 1454–1459
14. Randomised controlled trial of cardioprotective diet in patients with recent acute myocardial infarction: results of one year follow up. Singh RB, Rastogi SS, Verma R et al. *BMJ* 1992; 304: 1015–1019
15. Minnis RC, Haq IU, Jackson PR, Yeo WW Ramsay LE. Oily fish and fish oil supplements in the prevention of coronary heart disease. *J Hum Nutr Dietet* 1998; 11: 13–19
16. Shekelle RB, Missell L, Paul O, Shryock SM, Stamler J. Fish consumption and mortality from coronary heart disease. *N Engl J Med* 1985; 313: 820–821
17. Kromhout D, Bosschieter EB, de Lezenne Coulander C. The inverse relation between fish consumption and 20-year mortality from coronary heart disease. *N Engl J Med*. 1985; 312: 1205–1209
18. Norell SE, Ahlbom A, Feychting M, Pedersen NL. Fish consumption and mortality from coronary heart disease. *BMJ* 1986; 293: 426
19. Gramenzi A, Gentile A, Fasoli M, Negri E, Parazzini F, La Vecchia C. Association between certain foods and risk of acute myocardial infarction in women. *BMJ*. 1990; 300: 771–773
20. Ascherio A, Rimm EB, Stampfer MJ, Giovannucci EL, Willett WC. Dietary intake of marine n-3 fatty acids, fish intake, and the risk of coronary disease among men. N Engl J Med 1995; 332: 977–982
21. Yano K, Reed DM, Curb JD, Hankin JH, Albers JJ. Biological and dietary correlates of plasma lipids and lipoproteins among elderly Japanese men in Hawaii. *Arteriosclerosis*. 1986; 6: 422–433
22. Burr ML, Fehily AM, Gilbert JF et al. Effects of changes in fat, fish, and fibre intakes on death and myocardial reinfarction: Diet and reinfarction trial (DART). *Lancet* 1989; ii: 757–761
23. GISSI-Preventzione Investigators. Dietary supplementation with n-3 polyunsaturated fatty acids and vitamin E after myocardial infarction: results of the GISSI-Preventzione trial. *Lancet* 1999; 354: 447–455
24. Singh RB, Rastogi SS, Verma R et al. Randomised controlled trial of cardioprotective diet in patients with recent myocardial infarction: results of one year follow up. *BMJ* 1992; 304: 1015–1019
25. Saso Y, Kitamura K, Ysoshima A, Iwasaki HO, Takashima K, Doi K, Morita T. Rapid induction of atherosclerosis in rabbits. *Histology & Histopathology*. 1992; 7: 315–320
26. Fraser GE, Sabaté J, Beeson WL, Strahan M. A possible protective effect of nut consumption on risk of coronary heart disease. *Arch Intern Med* 1992; 152: 1416–1424
27. Hu FB, Stampfer MJ, Manson JE et al. Frequent nut consumption and risk of coronary heart disease in women: prospective cohort study. BMJ 1998; 317: 1341–1345
28. Sabaté J, Fraser GE, Burke K, Knutsen SF, Bennet H, Lindsted KD. Effects of walnuts on serum lipid levels and blood pressure in normal men. *N Engl J Med* 1993; 328: 603–607
29. Rimm EB, Ascherio A, Giovannucci E, Spiegelman D, Stampfer MJ, Willett WC. Vegetable, fruit, and cereal fiber intake and risk of coronary heart disease among men. JAMA 1996; 275: 447–451
30. Hankey GJ, Eikelboom JW. Homocysteine and vascular disease. *Lancet* 1999; 354: 407–413
31. Wilcken DE, Wilcken B. The pathogenesis of coronary artery disease. A possible role for methionine metabolism. *J clin Invest* 1976; 57: 1079–1082
32. Frosst P, Blom HJ, Milos R et al. A candidate genetic risk factor for vascular disease: a common mutation in methylenetetrahydrofolate reductase. *Nat Genet* 1995; 10: 111–113

33. Brattstrom L, Wilcken DEL, Ohrvik J, Brudin L. Common methylenetetrahydrofolate reductase gene mutation leads to hyperhomocysteinemia but not to vascular disease. *Circulation* 1998; 98: 2520–2526
34. Rimm EB, Willett WC, Hu FB et al. Folate and vitamin $B_6$from diet and supplements in relation to risk of coronary heart disease among women. *JAMA*. 1998; 279: 359–364
35. Homocysteine Lowering Trialists' Collaboration. Lowering blood homocysteine with folic acid based supplements: meta-analysis of randomised trials. *BMJ* 1998; 316: 894–898
36. Wilcken DEL, Wilcken B. The natural history of vascular disease in homocystinuria and the effects of treatment. J Inher Metab Dis 1997; 20: 295–300
37. Steinberg D, Pathasarathy S, Carew TE, Khoo JC, Witzum JL. Beyond cholesterol: modifications of low-density lipoprotein that increase its atherogenicity. *N Engl J Med* 1989; 320: 915–924
38. Steinberg D. Antioxidants in the prevention of human atherosclerosis: summary of the proceedings of a National Heart, Lung and Blood Institute Workshop: September 5–6, 1991, Bethesda, Maryland. *Circulation* 1992; 85: 2337–2344
39. Knekt P, Trunanen A, Javinen R, Seppanen R, Heliovaara M, Aromaa A. Antioxidant vitamin intake and coronary mortality in a longitudinal population study. *Am J Epidemiol* 1994; 139: 1180–1189
40. Manson JE, Stampfer MJ, Willett WC et al. A prospective study of vitamin C and incidence of coronary heart disease in women. *Circulation* 1992; 85: 865
41. Rimm EB, Stampfer MJ, Ascherio A, Giovannucci E, Colditz GA, Willett WC. Vitamin E consumption and the risk of coronary heart disease in men. *N Engl J Med* 1993; 328: 1450–1456
42. Enstrom JE, Kanim LE, Klein MA. Vitamin C intake and mortality among a sample of the United States population. *Epidemiology* 1992; 3: 194–202
43. Gale CR, Martyn CN, Winter PD, Cooper C. Vitamin C and risk of death from stroke and coronary heart disease in cohort of elderly people. *BMJ* 1995; 310: 1563–1566
44. Ness A, Egger M, Davey-Smith G. Role of antioxidant vitamins in prevention of cardiovascular diseases. *BMJ* 1999; 319: 577
45. Jha P, Flather M, Lonn E, Farkouh M, Yusuf S. The antioxidant vitamins and cardiovascular disease. *Ann Intern Med* 1995; 123: 860–872
46. Egger M, Schneider M, Davey-Smith G. *Meta-analysis* Spurious precision? Meta-analysis of observational studies. *BMJ* 1998; 316: 140–144
47. Rimm EB, Stampfer MJ, Ascherio A, Giovannucci E, Colditz GA, Willett WC. Vitamin E consumption and the risk of coronary heart disease in men. *N Engl. J Med* 1993; 328: 1450–1456
48. Stampfter MJ, Hennekens CH, Manson JE, Colditz GA, Rosner B, Willett WC. Vitamin E consumption and the risk of coronary heart disease in women. *N Engl J Med* 1993; 328: 1444–1449
49. Knekt P, Reunanen A, Jarvinen R, Seppanen R, Heliovaara M, Aromaa A. Antioxidant vitamin intake and coronary mortality in a longitudinal population study. *Am J of Epidemiol* 1994; 139: 1180–1189
50. Kushi LH, Folsom AR, Prineas RJ, Mink PJ, Wu Y, Bostick RM. Dietary antioxidant vitamins and death from coronary heart disease in postmenopausal women. N *Engl J Med* 1996; 334: 1156–1162
51. α-Tocopherol, β-Carotene Cancer Prevention Study Group. The effect of vitamin E and β-carotene on the incidence of lung cancer and other cancers in male smokers. *N Engl J Med* 1994; 330: 1029–1035
52. Rapola JM, Virtamo J, Haukka JK, Heinonen OP, Albanes D, Taylor PR et al. Effect of vitamin E and β-carotene on the incidence of angina pectoris: a randomized, double-blind, controlled trial. *JAMA* 1996; 275: 693–698
53. Rapola JM, Virtamo J, Ripatti S, Huttunen JK, Albanes D, Taylor PR et al. Randomised trial of tocopherol and carotene supplements on incidence of major coronary events in men with previous myocardial infarction. *Lancet* 1997; 349: 1715–1720

54. Stephens NG, Parsons A, Schofield PM, Kelly F, Cheeseman K, Mitchinson MJ et al. Randomised controlled trial of vitamin E in patients with coronary disease: Cambridge heart antioxidant study (CHAOS). *Lancet* 1996; 347: 781–786
55. The HOPE (Heart Outcomes Prevention Evaluation) Study Investigators. Effects of long-term vitamin E supplementation on cardiovascular events in 9541 high-risk persons. *N Engl J Med* (in press)
56. Steinberg D. Antioxidant Vitamins and Coronary Heart Disease. *N Engl J Med* 1993; 328: 1487–1489
57. Blackwelder WC, Yano K, Rhoads GG, Kagan A, Gordon T, Palesch Y. Alcohol and mortality: the Honolulu Heart Study. *Am J Med* 1980; 68: 164–169
58. Thun MJ, Peto R, Lopez AD et al. Alcohol consumption and mortality among middle-aged and elderly US adults. N *Engl J Med* 1997; 337: 1705–1714
59. Law M, Wald N. Why heart disease is low in France: the time lag explanation. *BMJ* 1999; 318: 1471–1480
60. Miettinen TA, Puska P, Gylling H, Vanhanen H, Vartiainen E. Reduction of serum cholesterol with sitostanol-ester margarine in a mildly hypercholesterolemic population. *N Engl J Med* 1995; 333: 1308–1312

12 The Scientific Basis for Fish Oil Supplementation in Rheumatoid Arthritis

Philip Calder

12.1 Introduction

Fish oil capsules are widely available in pharmacies, in supermarkets and by mail order. Many claims have been made about the "health giving" properties of such oils and there are articles and advertisements featuring them, appearing regularly in the popular press. They are often marketed as being "beneficial for arthritis", although it is probably not clear to the consumer why that should be. This chapter aims to present the scientific basis for the action of fish oils in rheumatoid arthritis and to give an overview of the evidence for benefits of fish oil in this disease. In order to do this it will be necessary to describe the amount and types of fat in the human diet, the components of the immune system and how they function to protect the host from infectious agents, and the immune dysfunction which occurs in rheumatoid arthritis.

12.2 Fatty Acids in the Human Diet

In Western countries an adult eats on average 75 to 150 g of fat each day and fat contributes 35 to 45% of dietary energy. By far the most important component of dietary fat in quantitative terms is triacylglycerol, which in the United Kingdom diet constitutes > 95% of dietary fat [1]. Other components of dietary fat include phospholipids, glycolipids, sterols and their esters and fat-soluble vitamins. Each triacylglycerol molecule is composed of three fatty acids esterified to a glycerol backbone; phospholipids, glycolipids and sterol esters also include fatty acids in their structure. Thus, fatty acids are a major constituent of dietary fat. Because of the range of foodstuffs consumed, the human diet contains a variety of fatty acids. Each fatty acid is a hydrocarbon chain of alternating -CH_2- units with a methyl group at one end and a carboxyl group at the other; it is the carboxyl group which is esterified to the glycerol backbone in triacylglycerols, phospholipids and glycolipids and to cholesterol in cholesterol esters. The most abundant fatty acids have straight chains of an even number of carbon atoms. The chain lengths vary from 4 in milk to 30 in some fish oils. Fatty acids may contain double bonds; these are then termed unsaturated fatty acids, as opposed to saturated fatty acids which do not contain any double bonds. The structure of some saturated and unsaturated fatty acids is

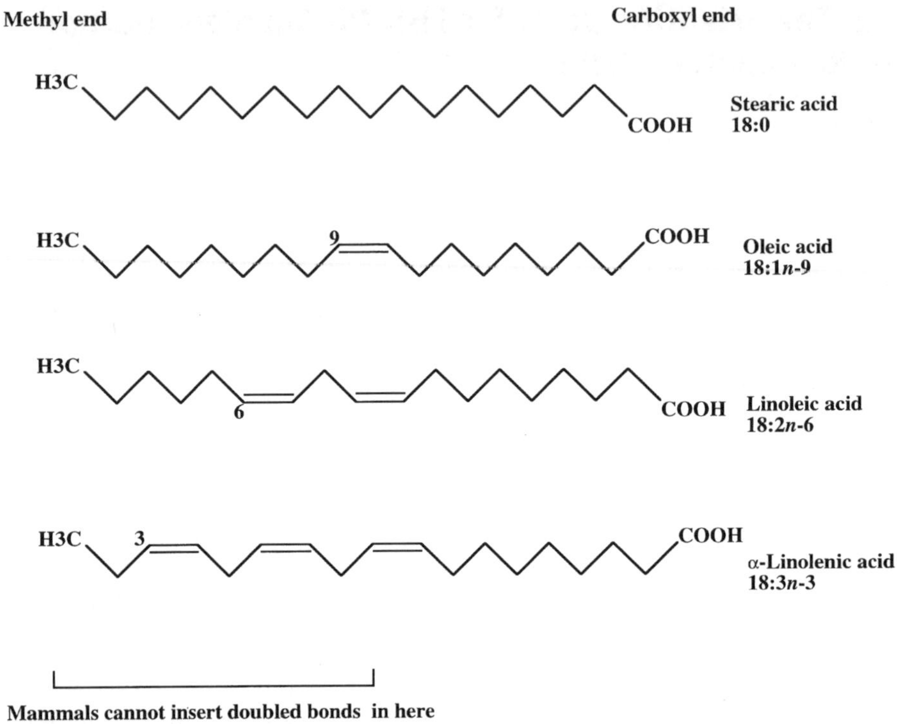

Fig. 1. The structure of a series of 18-carbon fatty acids. The position of insertion of double bonds is indicated, as is the basis for the *n*- nomenclature. Linoleic and α-linolenic acids cannot be synthesised in mammals because they cannot insert double bonds in the *n*-6 or *n*-3 positions

shown in Fig. 1. The number and position of the double bonds differs among different unsaturated fatty acids; if there are two or more double bonds the fatty acid is termed polyunsaturated. Most double bonds are in the *cis* form, although *trans* double bonds can be introduced through hydrogenation processes which may be natural (e.g. in the rumen of cattle) or part of the industrial processing of fats. It is the nature of the constituent fatty acids (their chain length and degree of unsaturation) which gives a fat its physical properties, specifically determining the temperature at which the fat will melt. Thus, fats which contain a high proportion of saturated fatty acids are often solid at room temperature (e.g. lard, butter) while fats which contain a high proportion of polyunsaturated fatty acids are liquid at room temperature (e.g. corn oil, sunflower oil).

Fatty acids have systematic names but most also have common names and are described by a shorthand nomenclature (Table 1). This nomenclature indicates the number of carbon atoms in the chain, the number of double bonds in the chain and the position of the first double bond from the methyl terminus of the chain (see Fig. 1). There are "rules" regarding the position of double bonds in unsaturated fatty acids; these are determined by the specificity of the enzymes

Table 1. Fatty acid nomenclature and sources

Systematic name	Trivial name	Shorthand notation	Sources
Decanoic	Capric	10:0	*de* novo synthesis; coconut oil
Dodecanoic	Lauric	12:0	*de* novo synthesis; coconut oil
Tetradecanoic	Myrsitic	14:0	*de* novo synthesis; milk
Hexadecanoic	Palmitic	16:0	*de* novo synthesis; milk; eggs; animal fats; meat; cocoa butter; palm oil (other vegetable oils contain lesser amounts); fish oils
Octadecanoic	Stearic	18:0	*de* novo synthesis; milk; eggs; animal fats; meat; cocoa butter
9-Hexadecenoic	Palmitoleic	16:1*n*-7	Desaturation of palmitic acid; fish oils
9-Octadecenoic	Oleic	18:1*n*-9	Desaturation of stearic acid; milk; eggs; animal fats; meat; cocoa butter; most vegetable oils, especially olive oil
9,12-Octadecadienoic	Linoleic	18:2*n*-6	Cannot be synthesised in mammals; some milks; eggs; animal fats; meat; most vegetable oils, especially corn, sunflower, safflower and soybean oils; green leaves
9,12,15-Octadecatrienoic	α-Linolenic	18:3*n*-3	Cannot be synthesised in mammals; green leaves; some vegetable oils especially rapeseed, soybean and linseed oils
6-9,12-Octadecatrienoic	γ-Linolenic	18:3*n*-6	Synthesised from linoleic acid; borage and evening primrose oils
11, 14,17-Eicosatrienoic	Mead	20:3*n*-9	Synthesised from oleic acid; indicator of essential fatty acid deficiency
8,11,14-Eicosatrienoic	Dihomo-γ-linolenic	20:3*n*-6	Synthesised from γ-linolenic acid
5,8,11,14-Eicosatetraenoic	Arachidonic	20:4*n*-6	Synthesised from linoleic acid via γ-linolenic and dihomo-γ-linolenic acids; meat
5,8,11,14,17-Eicosapentaenoic	Eicosapen-taenoic	20:5*n*-3	Synthesised from α-linolenic acid; fish oils
4,7,10,13,16,19-Docosahexaenoic	Docosahexa-enoic	22:6*n*-3	Synthesised from α-linolenic acid via eicosapentaenoic acid; fish oils

which insert those bonds into the hydrocarbon chain. It is the position of the first double bond in the hydrocarbon chain which is indicated by the *n*–7, *n*–9, *n*–6 or *n*–3 part of the shorthand notation for a fatty acid. Thus, an *n*–6 fatty acid has the first double bond on carbon number 6 counted from the methyl terminus and an *n*–3 fatty acid has the first double bond on carbon number 3 counted from the methyl terminus (see Fig. 1). Note that the *n*- notation is sometimes referred to as ω- or omega-.

Saturated fatty acids and most monounsaturated fatty acids can be made in mammalian tissues from non-fat precursors like glucose or amino acids, but this does not usually occur in humans eating a Western diet since the consumption of fat in general, and of saturated and monounsaturated fatty acids in particular, is high. However, mammals cannot insert double bonds before carbon number 9 in oleic acid. Thus, mammals cannot convert oleic acid (18:1*n*–9) into linoleic acid (18:2*n*–6). The enzyme which does this conversion is called Δ^{12}-desaturase and this is found only in plants. Likewise, mammals cannot convert linoleic acid into α-linolenic acid (18:3*n-3*). The enzyme which does this is called Δ^{15}-desaturase and again this is found only in plants. Because these two fatty acids cannot be made by mammals they are termed essential fatty acids. Also because mammalian tissues do not contain the Δ^{15}-desaturase they cannot interconvert *n*-6 and *n-3* fatty acids. Plant tissues and plant oils tend to be rich sources of linoleic and α-linolenic acids. For example, linoleic acid contributes over 50% and often up to 80% of the fatty acids found in corn, sunflower, safflower and soybean oils. Rapeseed and soybean oils are also good sources of α-linolenic acid since this fatty acid contributes between 5 and 15% of the fatty acids present. However, the richest source of α-linolenic acid is linseed oil. α-linolenic acid contributes up to 60% of the fatty acids in linseed oil. In North America linseed oil is known as flaxseed oil. The major fatty acids in the diet of adults in the United Kingdom are medium and long chain saturated fatty acids, especially myristic, palmitic and stearic, the monounsaturated fatty acid oleic, and the polyunsaturated fatty acids linoleic and α-linolenic. Over the period since 1970 the absolute consumption of saturated fatty acids in the United Kingdom has declined by 40%, while the consumption of monounsaturated fatty acids has declined by 30% [1]. The consumption of polyunsaturated fatty acids increased by 25% over this period of time [1]. This was largely the result of increased consumption of linoleic acid which became generally available in margarines and cooking oils. According to the Dietary and Nutritional Survey of British Adults the daily diet of the average adult male in the United Kingdom contains 42 g saturated fatty acids, 31 g monounsaturated fatty acids and 15.8 g polyunsaturated fatty acids [1]. The main polyunsaturated fatty acid in the diet is linoleic acid (intake is approximately 13.8 g/day for adult males) with α-linolenic acid contributing approximately 2 g/day [1, 2]. Adult females show a similar pattern of fatty acid consumption to males but the absolute amounts of each type of fatty acid consumed are about 70% of those consumed by males [1, 2].

Once consumed in the diet linoleic acid can be converted via γ-linolenic (18:3*n*–6) and dihomo-γ-linolenic (20:3*n*–6) acids to arachidonic acid (20:4*n*–6) by the pathway outlined in Fig. 2. γ-Linolenic acid is a constituent of borage oil (also known as starflower oil) and evening primrose oil, but intake of this fatty acid from habitual diets is very low, probably <20 mg/day. There are no estimates of the intake of arachidonic acid from the United Kingdom diet, but estimates from Australia and the United States suggest intakes of between 50 and 300 mg/day for adults [3–5]. Using the same pathway (Fig. 2) dietary α-linolenic acid can be converted into eicosapentaenoic acid (EPA; 20:5*n-3*) and docosahexaenoic acid (DHA; 22:6*n-3*). The intake of longer chain polyunsaturated fatty acids is not clearly known but it appears that the average adult in the United

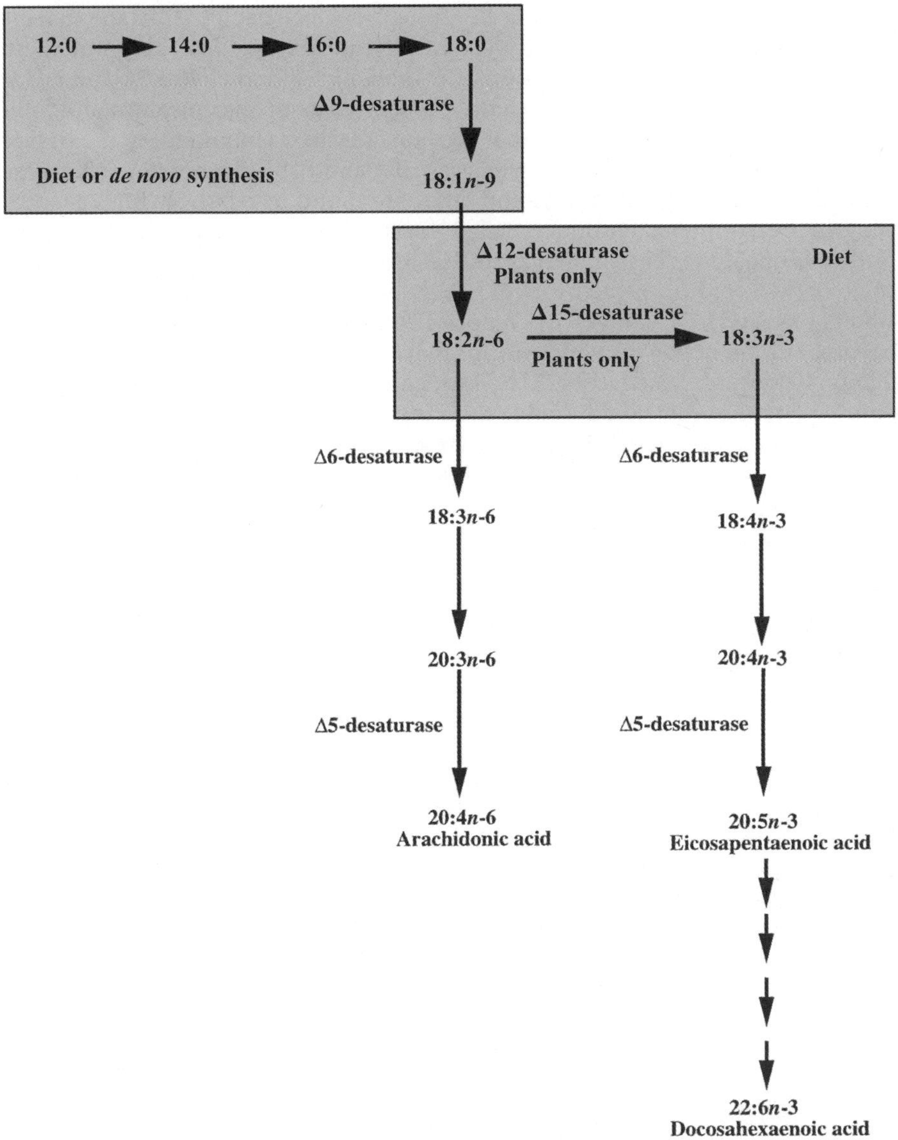

Fig. 2. The pathways for synthesis of polyunsaturated fatty acids. Saturated fatty acids and oleic acid can be synthesised in mammalian tissues, but linoleic and α-linolenic acids cannot since mammals do not have the enzymes required (plants do). Once consumed in the diet linoleic and α-linolenic acids can be metabolised to longer chain, more unsaturated derivatives

Kingdom consumes about 250 mg EPA plus DHA per day [1, 2]. Many marine plants, especially the unicellular algae in phytoplankton, also carry out chain elongation and further desaturation of α-linolenic acid to yield EPA and DHA. It is the formation of these long chain *n-3* fatty acids by marine algae and their transfer through the food chain, that accounts for their abundance in the tissues of some marine mammals (e.g. whales, seals) and fish (e.g. herring, mackerel, tuna; known as "oily fish"). EPA and DHA are found in relatively high proportions in the commercial products called "fish oils" which are a preparation of the body oils of cold water fish; EPA and DHA are also found in high proportions in the oils extracted from the livers of other species of fish which live in warmer waters (e.g. cod). EPA and DHA comprise 20 to 30% of the fatty acids in a typical preparation of fish oil, which means that a one gram fish oil capsule provides 200 to 300 mg of these fatty acids. Thus, an adult in the United Kingdom consuming a typical diet could double their intake of long chain n-3 fatty acids by consuming a single one gram fish oil capsule per day. In contrast, consumption of a single portion of oily fish can provide as much as two or three grams of long chain n-3 fatty acids [2]. Note however, that in the absence of significant consumption of oily fish, α-linolenic acid is the major dietary n-3 fatty acid.

12.3 The Immune System

12.3.1 What is the Immune System and How Does it Work?

The immune system acts to protect the host from infectious agents which exist in the environment (bacteria, viruses, fungi, parasites) and from other noxious insults. The immune system has two functional divisions: the innate (or natural) immune system and the acquired (also termed specific or adaptive) immune system. Both components of immunity involve various blood-borne factors and cells (Table 2). These cells are generally termed leukocytes (or white blood cells).

Table 2. Components of innate and acquired immunity

	Innate	Acquired
Physicochemical barriers	Skin	Cutaneous and mucosal immune systems
	Mucous membranes Lysozyme Stomach acid Commensal bacteria	Antibodies in mucosal secretions
Circulating molecules	Complement	Antibodies
Cells	Granulocytes Monocytes/macrophages Natural killer cells	Lymphocytes (T and B)
Soluble mediators	Macrophage-derived cytokines	Lymphocyte-derived cytokines

Leukocytes fall into two broad categories: phagocytes (which include granulocytes [neutrophils, basophils, eosinophils], monocytes and macrophages) and lymphocytes. Lymphocytes are further subdivided into T lymphocytes, B lymphocytes and natural killer cells. T lymphocytes are further divided into helper T cells (these are distinguished by the presence of the molecule CD4 on their surface) and cytotoxic T cells (these are distinguished by the presence of CD8 on their surface). The cells of the immune system are found circulating in the bloodstream, organised into lymphoid organs such as the thymus, spleen and lymph nodes or dispersed in other locations around the body. All cells of the immune system originate in bone marrow.

Innate immunity is the first line of defence against infectious agents. It is present prior to exposure to pathogens and its activity is not enhanced by such exposures. This component of immunity includes:

- the skin;
- other physiochemical barriers to entry of pathogens such as the mucous lining of the respiratory, gastrointestinal and genitourinary tracts, lysozyme in tears, acid in the stomach, and commensal bacteria in the gastrointestinal tract;
- phagocytic cells and natural killer cells in the blood and tissues;
- blood-borne chemicals such as complement, acute phase proteins and cytokines produced by macrophages (Table 2).

Innate immunity is concerned with preventing entry of infectious agents into the body and, if they do enter, with their rapid elimination. Elimination can occur by:

- direct destruction of pathogens by complement, by toxic chemicals, such as superoxide radicals and hydrogen peroxide released by phagocytes, or by toxic proteins released by natural killer cells;
- engulfing pathogens by the process of phagocytosis (this is what phagocytes do; phagocytosis is made more efficient by coating the invading pathogen with host proteins like complement or antibodies) and their subsequent destruction.

Acquired immunity involves the specific recognition of molecules on an invading pathogen which distinguish it as being foreign to the host (these are called antigens). The recognition of antigens is by antibodies (produced by B lymphocytes) and by T lymphocytes (Table 2). The acquired immune system includes a component of memory, such that if the antigen is encountered again (i.e. there is re-infection) the response is faster and stronger than the initial response. This is the basis of vaccination. Although the immune system as a whole can recognise tens of thousands of antigens, each lymphocyte can recognise only one antigen and so the number of lymphocytes specific for a particular antigen must be very low. However, when an antigen is encountered it binds to the small number of lymphocytes which recognise it and causes them to divide so as to increase the number of cells which are capable of mounting a response to the antigen; this is the process termed lymphocyte proliferation. B lymphocytes proliferate and mature into antibody-producing cells (plasma cells) and T lymphocytes proliferate and are able to directly destroy virally-infected cells (cytotoxic T lymphocytes) or control the activity of other cells involved in the response (helper T cells). The B lymphocyte response to antigen is termed humoural immunity and the T cell response is termed cell-mediated immunity.

12.3.2 Communication Within the Immune System: Cytokines

Communication within the acquired immune system and between the innate and acquired systems is brought about by direct cell-to-cell contact involving adhesion molecules and by the production of chemical messengers which send signals from one cell to another (Fig. 3). Chief among these chemical messengers are proteins called cytokines which can act to regulate the activity of the cell which produced the cytokine or of other cells. Each cytokine can have multiple activities on different cell types. Cytokines act by binding to specific receptors

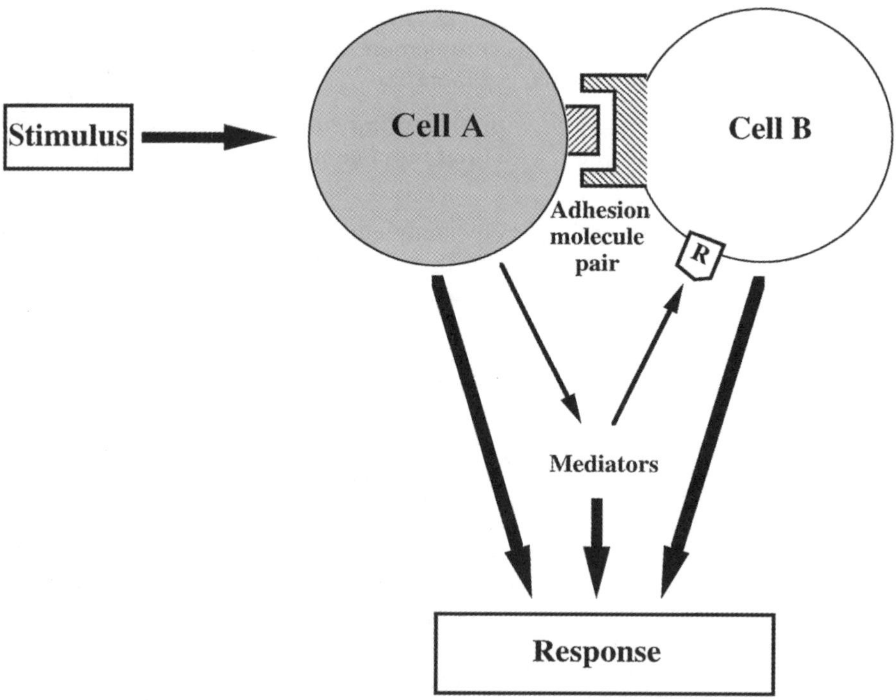

Fig. 3. Schematic representation of how immune cells interact to give a co-ordinated response to a stimulus. There may be direct cell-to-cell interaction mediated by proteins (e.g. adhesion molecules) on the surface of the two interacting cells and/or there may be production of chemical messengers (i.e. mediators) by one cell type which affect the activities of the second cell type. The specificity of action of most mediators is determined by the presence of receptors (R) on the surface of target cells

on the cell surface and thereby induce changes in growth, development, or activity of the target cell.

Tumour necrosis factor (TNF)-α, interleukin (IL)-1 and IL-6 are among the most important cytokines produced by monocytes and macrophages. These cytokines activate neutrophils, monocytes and macrophages to initiate bacterial and tumour cell killing, increase adhesion molecule expression on the surface of neutrophils and endothelial cells, stimulate T and B lymphocyte proliferation, up-regulate major histocompatibility antigens (these are involved in the presentation of antigen to T lymphocytes) and initiate the production of other pro-inflammatory cytokines (e.g. TNF induces production of IL-1 and IL-6, and IL-1 induces production of IL-6). Thus, TNF, IL-1 and IL-6 are mediators of both natural and acquired immunity and are an important link between them. In addition, these cytokines mediate the systemic effects of inflammation such as fever, weight loss and acute phase protein synthesis in the liver. Production of appropriate amounts of TNF, IL-1 and IL-6 is clearly beneficial in response to infection, but inappropriate or overproduction can be dangerous and these cytokines, especially TNF, are implicated in causing some of the pathological responses which occur in inflammatory conditions [6].

Helper T lymphocytes can be sub-divided according to the pattern of cytokines they produce (Fig. 4). It is believed that helper T cells which have not previously encountered antigen produce mainly IL-2 upon initial encounter with antigen. These cells may differentiate into a population sometimes referred to as Th0 cells which differentiate further into either Th1 or Th2 cells (Fig. 4). This differentiation is regulated by cytokines: IL-12 and interferon-γ (IFN-γ) promote the development of Th1 cells while IL-4 promotes the development of Th2 cells (Fig. 4). Th1 and Th2 themselves have relatively restricted profiles of cytokine production: Th1 cells produce IL-2 and IFN-γ which activate macrophages, natural killer cells and cytotoxic T lymphocytes and are the principal effectors of cell-mediated immunity. Interactions with bacteria, viruses and fungi tend to induce Th1 activity. Since Th1 cytokines activate monocytes and macrophages, these cytokines may be regarded as pro-inflammatory. Th2 cells produce IL-4, which stimulates immunoglobulin E production, IL-5, an eosinophil activating factor, and IL-10, which together with IL-4 suppresses cell-mediated immunity (Fig. 4). Th2 cells are responsible for defence against helminthic parasites which is due to immunoglobulin E-mediated activation of mast cells and basophils. Because Th2 cytokines suppress Th1 responses, these cytokines may be regarded as anti-inflammatory.

12.3.3 Inflammation

Inflammation is the body's immediate response to infection or injury. It is typified by redness, swelling, heat and pain. These symptoms occur as a result of increased blood flow, increased permeability across blood capillaries which permits large molecules (e.g. complement, antibodies, cytokines) to leave the bloodstream and cross the endothelial wall and increased movement of leukocytes from the bloodstream into the surrounding tissue. Thus, inflammation is part of the normal, innate immune response.

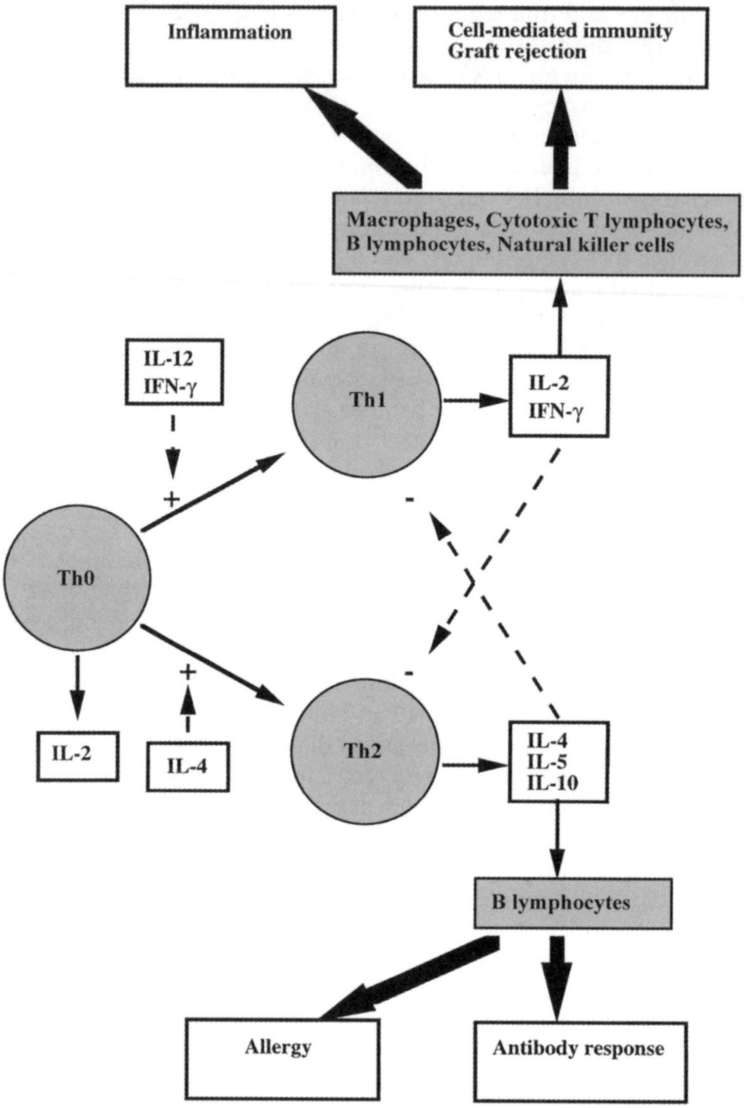

Fig. 4. The differentiation of helper T lymphocytes and their involvement in immune responses and in disease processes. According to the cytokine mileu, helper T lymphocytes can differentiate towards the Th1 phenotype or towards the Th2 phenotype. The presence of bacterial, viral or fungul infections promotes differentiation along the Th1 path whereas the presence of parasitic infections promotes differentiation along the Th2 pathway. Th1 cells produce interleukin-2 (IL-2) and interferon-γ (IFN-γ). These activate macrophages, cytotoxic T lymphocytes, natural killer cells and B lymphocytes to elicit cell-mediated immune responses and graft rejection. Th2 cells produce IL-4, IL-5 and IL-10. IL-4 promotes the production of immunoglobulin E by B lymphocytes and IL-5 enhances eosinophil activity. Th1 cytokines inhibit the development of Th2 cells while Th2 cytokines inhibit the development of Th1 cells. The Th1 response is involved in chronic inflammation while the Th2 response is involved in allergic reactions

12.3.4 Integration of the Immune Response

The innate and acquired immune responses are integrated according to the direct cell-to-cell and cytokine interactions which result from the presence of a particular stimulus. The innate response, including its inflammatory component, responds initially to the stimulus, acting directly to eliminate it by the activities of complement, phagocytosis etc. Cytokines produced by the cells involved in the innate response, especially monocytes and macrophages, will regulate this response and also act systemically on the liver to promote acute phase protein synthesis, on skeletal muscle and adipose tissue to promote proteolysis and lipolysis, respectively (this is believed to be the body's way of providing fuels to the immune system), and on the brain to reduce appetite and induce fever (Fig. 5). These cytokines will also interact with T lymphocytes. Antigen-presenting cells which include activated monocytes and macrophages will present antigen to T lymphocytes and so the acquired immune response will be triggered (Fig. 5). Now there will be a cell-mediated response to the antigen. T lymphocytes will produce cytokines which will regulate the activity of the cells involved

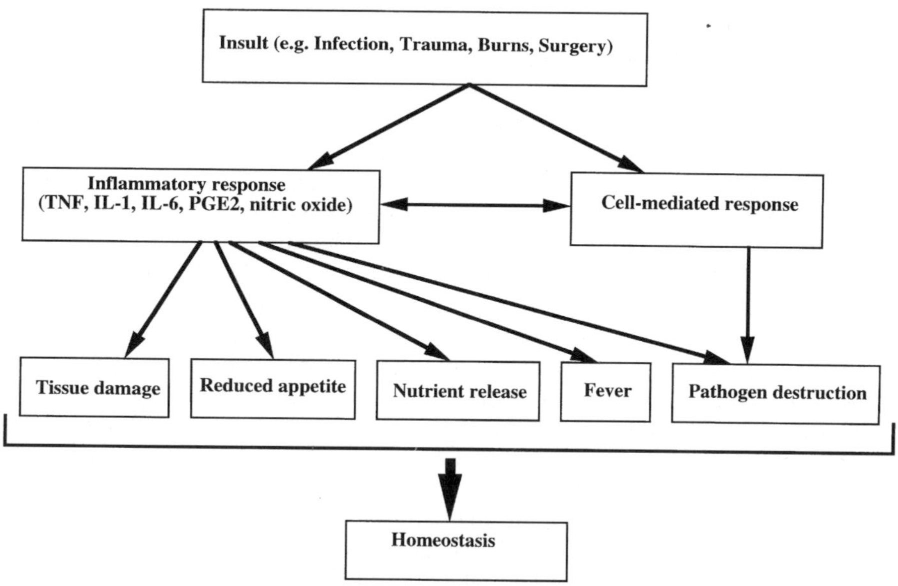

Fig. 5. Schematic representation of the immune response to an insult. An immunological insult may be infectious in nature or may be related to injury. The insult activates the inflammatory response. The presence of antigen and/or certain cytokines activates the cell-mediated immune response. The mediators produced as part of the inflammatory response induce systemic effects (e.g. reduced appetite, release of stored nutrients, fever), which are believed to play a role in optimising the host response. The inflammatory and cell-mediated responses together lead to pathogen destruction. In the course of the response there may be some damage to host tissues. Ultimately the source of the insult is eliminated and the system returns to homeostasis

in the innate response (monocytes, macrophages, natural killer cells), promote the proliferation of B and T lymphocytes and promote antibody production by B lymphocytes. By virtue of the integrated innate and acquired responses the source of the antigen should be eliminated and a component of immunological memory will remain (Fig. 5).

12.3.5 The Immune System in Health and Disease

Clearly a well functioning immune system is essential to health. It serves to protect the host from the effects of ever present pathogenic organisms. Cells of the immune system also have a role in identifying and eliminating cancer cells. There are however some detrimental effects of the immune system:

1. In the course of its activity to recognise and eliminate foreign antigens, the immune system is responsible for the rejection of transplanted tissues.
2. In some individuals the immune system appears to be able to recognise host antigens. As a result, an immune response to host tissues is generated and this leads to tissue damage. This is the characteristic of so-called chronic inflammatory or autoimmune diseases. Such diseases are linked to genes coding for proteins involved in antigen presentation or recognition such as the major histocompatibility class II proteins and the T-cell receptor; thus there is a genetic predisposition to these diseases. These diseases are typified by an ongoing chronic inflammation involving the pro-inflammatory cytokines produced by monocytes and macrophages and by a dysregulated Th1 lymphocyte response. Examples of this type of disease include type-1 diabetes (IFN-γ expression correlates with β-cell destruction), psoriasis (IFN-γ but not IL-4 is found in the lesions), multiple sclerosis (T cells from patients produce IFN-γ but not IL-4) and rheumatoid arthritis (see below).
3. The immune system of some individuals can become sensitised to usually benign antigens from the environment and can respond inappropriately to them. Such antigens can include components of foods or of so-called allergens (e.g. cat or dog fur, house dust mite, some pollens), such that this response can lead to allergies, asthma and related atopic diseases. Although these diseases are often termed chronic inflammatory diseases they have a different immune basis from the diseases described above, although again they are typified by inappropriate recognition of and/or responses to antigens. However, atopic diseases are characterised by a dysregulated Th2 lymphocyte response such that excessive amounts of IL-4, IL-5 and IL-10 are found. IL-10 suppresses the Th1 response, IL-4 stimulates immunoglobulin E production by B lymphocytes (immunoglobulin E promotes histamine release from mast cells), and IL-4 and IL-5 activate eosinophils which are involved in the persistent inflammation which is a component of these diseases.
4. The immune system becomes activated as a result of trauma and surgery. This response is characterised by excess production of the pro-inflammatory cytokines and if it persists it can damage organs causing their failure leading to complications and sometimes death.

These immune dysfunctions are each characterised by the same set of events of characterise normal immune responses:

- recognition of the antigen/insult;
- inflammatory response (cellular activation and the release of chemoattractants, cytokines, eicosanoids, reactive species [e.g. superoxide radicals] and growth factors);
- chemotaxis of leukocytes towards the site of immune activity;
- upregulation of adhesion molecules promoting movement of leukocytes from the bloodstream to the sub-endothelial space;
- persistent cellular activation characterised by production of cytokines and other mediators (chronic inflammation);
- elimination of antigen/insult followed by reversal of cellular activation (if the immune response is successful) or tissue damage (in the case of inflammatory diseases).

12.4 Rheumatoid Arthritis

Rheumatoid arthritis (RA) is a common disease in humans with a prevalence of about 1 in 100 world-wide [7]; it is more common in women than in men [7]. RA is a chronic inflammatory or autoimmune disease. It is characterised by infiltration of activated T lymphocytes, macrophages and plasma cells (B lymphocytes which have differentiated into antibody secreting cells) into the synovial joints. This leads to progressive destruction of cartilage and bone, most likely due in part to cytokine induction of destructive enzymes such as matrix metalloproteinases. RA is also characterised by signs of systemic inflammation, such as elevated concentrations of acute phase proteins.

Genetic studies have linked vulnerability to and severity of RA to genes in the major histocompatibility class II locus [8]; in humans these proteins are called human leukocyte antigen class II (HLA). Specifically, RA is associated with a region in the genes encoding HLA-DR4 and HLA-DR1 [8]. Since the function of HLA-DR is to present antigen to helper T lymphocytes, this genetic association indicates a role for T cells in the disease. It seems that there is presentation of host antigen to T cells, which are driven along the Th1 path of differentiation thus promoting a pro-inflammatory response. The host antigen to which T cells react is not known but candidates include collagen type II, other cartilage proteins and heat shock protein 70. Despite this apparently central role of T cells in RA, there are low levels of T cell-derived cytokines in the synovial joints of RA patients and T-cell proliferation rates are low. This has been taken to indicate that T lymphocytes are not important in perpetuating the disease [9]. However, T lymphocytes normally play a key role in driving immune responses and they are central to animal models of autoimmune diseases including those for arthritis. Thus, T lymphocytes are likely to play a role in both RA induction and in its perpetuation.

Synovial biopsies from patients with RA contain high levels of pro-inflammatory cytokines including TNF-α, IL-1β, IL-6, IL-8 and granulocyte/macrophage-colony stimulating factor (GM-CSF) [10]. Synovial cells cultured *ex vivo* produce TNF-α, IL-1β, IL-6, IL-8 and GM-CSF for extended periods of time without additional stimulus [10]. If the action of TNF-α is blocked, for example by adding an anti-TNF-α antibody the production of the other cytokines is reduced, while if the action of IL-1 is blocked by adding IL-1 receptor antagonist (IL-1ra) the production of the other cytokines, except for TNF-α, is blocked [10]. This indicates a cascade of pro-inflammatory cytokines and suggests that blocking TNF-α will diminish the actions of many other pro-inflammatory mediators and so might be a therapeutic target.

The actions of pro-inflammatory cytokines are antagonised by anti-inflammatory cytokines such as IL-4, IL-10, transforming growth factor-β (TGF-β) and by cytokine inhibitors such as IL-1ra and soluble TNF receptors. Synovial biopsies from rheumatoid joints contain abundant amounts of TGF-β, IL-10 (but not IL-4, suggesting that the T cells involved in RA are of the Th1 type), IL-1ra and soluble TNF receptors [10]. Thus, the inflamed synovial joint contains excessive amounts of both pro- and anti-inflammatory mediators, but given the ongoing inflammatory state and what is known from animal models of arthritis, it appears that RA is characterised by an imbalance between pro- and anti-inflammatory cytokines and, most likely, between Th1 and Th2 cytokines.

12.5 Eicosanoids: The Link Between Fatty Acids and the Immune System

12.5.1 Eicosanoid Synthesis

Eicosanoids are a second group of chemical messengers which act within the immune system. They are synthesised from fatty acids, in particular dihomo-γ-linolenic, arachidonic and eicosapentaenoic acids. Eicosanoids include prostaglandins (PG), thromboxanes, leukotrienes (LT), lipoxins, hydroperoxyeicosatetraenoic acids and hydroxy-eicosatetraenoic acids. The fatty acid precursor for eicosanoid synthesis is released from cell membrane phospholipids, usually by the action of phospholipase A_2 activated in response to a cellular stimulus. Because the membranes of most cells contain large amounts of arachidonic acid, compared with dihomo-γ-linolenic acid and EPA, arachidonic acid is usually the principal precursor for eicosanoid synthesis and gives rise to the a particular family (called the 2-series) PG and thromboxanes and a particular family (called the 4-series) LT (Fig. 6). PG and thromboxanes are produced by the cyclooxygenase enzymes (COX). There are two isoforms of COX: COX-1 is a constitutive enzyme and COX-2 is induced in immune cells as a result of stimulation and is responsible for the markedly elevated production of PG which occurs upon cellular activation. Non-steroidal anti-inflammatory drugs (NSAIDs) act by inhibition of COX (Fig. 6).

LT and related compounds are produced by lipoxygenase enzymes (LOX) of which there are three types, each of which has a particular cellular distribution: 5-LOX is found in mast cells, monocytes, macrophages and granulocytes, 12-LOX is found in platelets and some epithelial cells and 15-LOX is found in young myeloid cells and some epithelial cells.

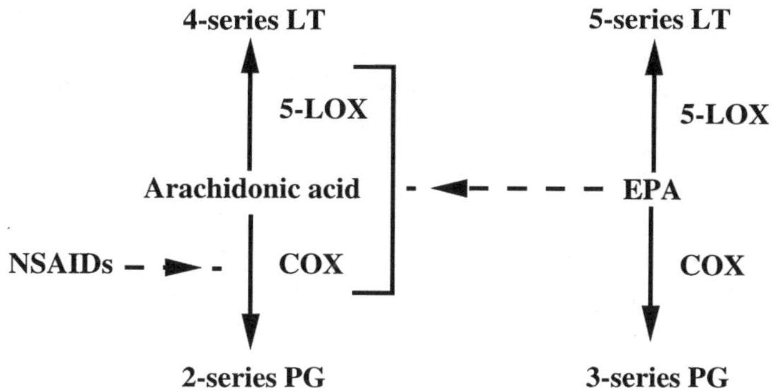

Fig. 6. Eicosanoid synthesis from arachidonic and eicosapentaenoic acids. Metabolism of arachidonic acid yields 2-series prostaglandins (PG) and 4-series leukotrienes (LT). The cyclooxygenase enzyme is inhibited by NSAIDs. When available through the diet, EPA partly replaces arachidonic acid in cell membranes, thereby decreasing the amount of substrate available for synthesis of 2-series PG and 4-series LT. EPA is a substrate for COX and 5-lipoxygenase (LOX) and gives rise to 3-series PG and 5-series LT

12.5.2 Roles for Eicosanoids in Inflammation and Immunity

PG are involved in modulating the intensity and duration of inflammatory and immune responses. PGE_2 has a number of pro-inflammatory effects including induction of fever and erythema, increasing vascular permeability and vasodilation and enhancing pain and oedema caused by other agents such as bradykinin and histamine. PGE_2 inhibits production of TNF-α, IL-1, IL-6, IL-2 and IFN-γ; thus in these respects PGE_2 is anti-inflammatory. PGE_2 does not affect the production of the Th2 cytokines IL-4 and IL-10 but promotes immunoglobulin E production by B lymphocytes.

LTB_4 increases vascular permeability, enhances local blood flow, is a potent chemotactic agent for leukocytes, induces release of lysosomal enzymes, enhances generation of reactive oxygen species and inhibits lymphocyte proliferation. 4-series LT also regulate production of pro-inflammatory cytokines; for example LTB_4 enhances production of TNF, IL-1 and IL-6.

12.5.3 Eicosanoids and RA

Both COX-1 and COX-2 expression are increased in the synovium of RA patients [11], and in the joint tissues in rat models of arthritris [11]. PGE_2, LTB_4, 5-HETE and also platelet activating factor, another phospholipid-derived inflammatory mediator, are found in the synovial fluid of patients with active RA [12]. In addition to the activities outlined above, PGE_2 promotes production of matrix metalloproteinases [13] and stimulates bone resorption [14]. The efficacy of NSAIDs in RA indicates the importance of the pro-inflammatory COX pathway products in the pathophysiology of the disease. However, although these drugs provide immediate relief of pain and stiffness by inhibiting joint inflammation, they do not influence the course of the disease. Second line drugs termed slow-acting antirhematic drugs (SAARDs) have a delayed action and can alter the course of RA. In general these drugs do not interfere with eicosanoid synthesis. An exception is the corticosteroids which have a range of potent anti-inflammatory effects including inhibition of phospholipase A_2, the enzyme responsible for release of arachidonic acid from membrane phospholipids prior to eicosanoid synthesis, and of COX-2 expression [29]. Both NSAIDs and SAARDs have side effects which limit the length of time that they can be used for.

12.5.4 Fish Oil and Eicosanoids

Feeding animals or humans increased amounts of fish oil results in a decrease in the amount of arachidonic acid in the membranes of most cells in the body, including those involved in inflammation such as monocytes, macrophages, neutrophils and lymphocytes. This means that there is less substrate available for synthesis of eicosanoids from arachidonic acid. Furthermore, EPA and DHA competitively inhibit the oxygenation of arachidonic acid by COX. Thus, fish oil feeding results in a decreased capacity of immune cells to synthesise eicosanoids from arachidonic acid (e.g. PGE_2 and LTB_4). In addition, EPA is able to act as a substrate for both COX and 5-LOX (Fig. 6), giving rise to derivatives which have a different structure from those produced from arachidonic acid (i.e. 3-series PG and thromboxanes and 5-series LT). Thus, the EPA-induced suppression in the production of arachidonic-acid derived eicosanoids is mirrored by an elevation in the production of EPA-derived eicosanoids [15, 16]. The eicosanoids produced from EPA are often less biologically potent than the analogues synthesised from arachidonic acid, although the full range of biological activities of these compounds has not been investigated. LTB_5 is only about 10% as potent as a chemotactic agent and in promoting lysosomal enzyme release as LTB_4 [17]. LTB_5 can partially inhibit LTB_4-mediated superoxide formation and chemotaxis [18].

12.6 Effects of Fish Oil on Immune Function

The effect of dietary *n-3* polyunsaturated fatty acids on production of eicosanoids derived from arachidonic acid (see above) suggests that fish oil should exert anti-inflammatory effects by decreasing the production of pro-inflammatory 2-series PG and 4-series LT. This effect should in turn alter other cellular functions such as the production of pro-inflammatory cytokines by monocytes and macrophages and by Th1 lymphocytes. A large number of studies on the effects of *n-3* fatty acids on immune function have now been published. These studies have examined the effects of *n-3* fatty acids added to isolated cells in culture (i.e. *in vitro* studies), the effects of feeding animals or humans diets containing increased amounts of *n-3* fatty acids on the functions of cells subsequently studied in culture (*ex vivo* studies), and the effects of feeding animals diets containing increased amounts of *n-3* fatty acids on *in vivo* measures of immune function such as responses to injected antigen or foreign cells (*in vivo* studies). Cell culture studies are useful to identify the potential effects of nutrients and to investigate their mechanisms of action. However, they represent a rather unphysiological setting since they use purified cells away from their normal environment and isolated from the interactions and signals that they would receive *in vivo*. *Ex vivo* studies can reveal the potential effects of nutrients *in vivo*, but again they usually involve the culture of isolated cells often for several days in an unphysiological setting, which might act to mask the effects of the nutrient under study. In contrast, *in vivo* studies reveal the response of the entire immune system to challenge; the concentration of antibodies or cytokines in the plasma can be measured, as can responses like fever, and swelling. Although there have been many studies of the impact of fish oil on inflammation and immunity, there are relatively few of these *in vivo* investigations, especially in humans. The studies of fish oil and inflammation and immunity have been reviewed in great detail a number of times recently [19–27], and need only be summarised here. With regard to RA the principal effects of fish oil, in addition to decreased production of arachidonic acid-derived eicosanoids, appear to be:

- decreased production of pro-inflammatory cytokines (TNF-α, IL-1 and IL-6) by monocytes and macrophages (demonstrated in some, but not all, studies in animals and humans);
- decreased lymphocyte reactivity and production of Th1-type cytokines (IL-2 and IFN-γ);
- decreased production of platelet activating factor;
- decreased production of reactive oxygen species (e.g. superoxide radicals) (demonstrated in some studies);
- decreased expression of major histocompatibility class II molecules;
- decreased expression of adhesion molecules on endothelial cells and leukocytes and decreased cell-to-cell binding;
- decreased chemotaxis of monocytes and neutrophils.

It should be mentioned that not all studies which have been performed agree and that there are some differences among animal studies and between some animal and human studies. Nevertheless, a large number of studies now support the idea that fish oil exerts a range of immunological effects. Thus, given the effects listed above, fish oil would be expected to diminish the recognition of and response to host antigen, decrease movement of leukocytes towards sites of inflammatory activity, decrease binding of leukocytes to endothelial cells and their movement from the bloodstream to the sub-endothelial space and decrease cellular activation and the release of chemoattractants, cytokines, eicosanoids and reactive species.

12.7
Fish Oil Intervention in Rheumatoid Arthritis

As outlined above, RA is a typical chronic inflammatory disease characterised by infiltration of leukocytes into the synovial joints, their activation and production of pro-inflammatory cytokines (TNF-α, IL-1, IL-6, IL-8), eicosanoids (PGE_2, LTB_4), superoxide radicals, proteinases and so on and subsequent joint destruction (Fig. 7). Increasing the consumption of fish oil results in decreased production of arachidonic acid derived eicosanoids, increased production of less potent EPA-derived eicosanoids, and decreased production of pro-inflammatory cytokines, platelet activating factor, and superoxide radicals. Thus, fish oil should act in RA to decrease the production of pro-inflammatory mediators which directly or indirectly contribute to joint destruction and to the systemic effects of the disease. In addition, it appears that fish oil decreases adhesion

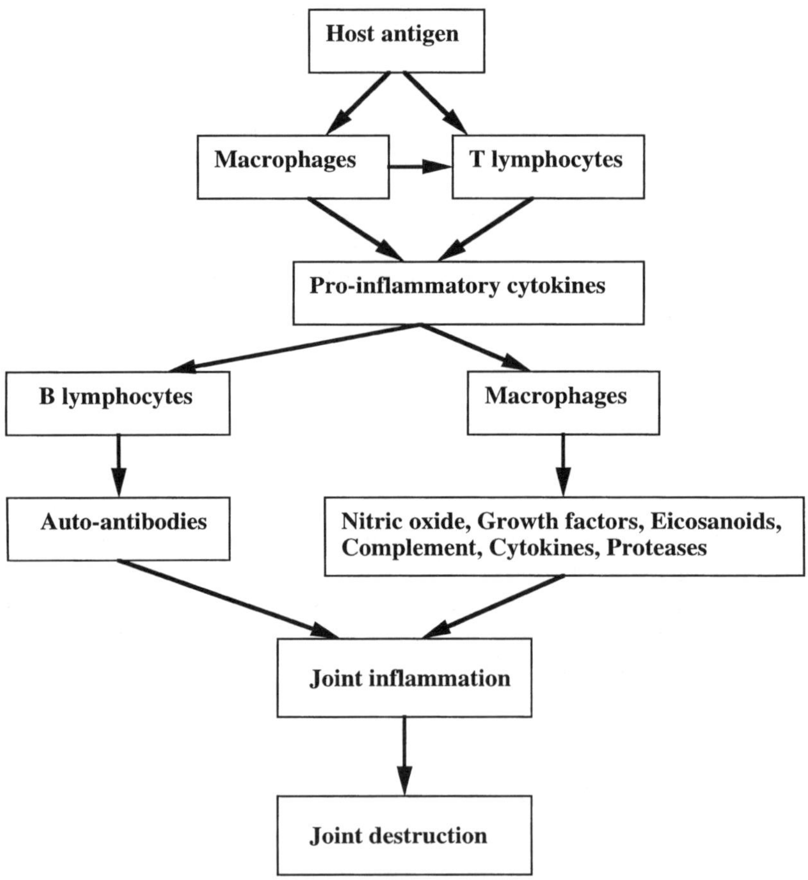

Fig. 7. The immunolgical response to host antigen in rheumatoid arthritis. The sustained production of inflammatory mediators leads to joint destruction

molecule expression on both endothelial cells and leukocytes and so might act to decrease leukocyte infiltration into the inflamed joint. Using a murine model of arthritis (type II collagen-induced arthritis) Leslie et al. [28] compared the effects of feeding diets rich in *n*–6 or *n-3* polyunsaturated fatty acids (corn oil vs. fish oil). The mice were fed the diets for 26 days and were then injected with type II collagen. They were retained on the diets for a further 80 days. Time of onset of arthritis was earlier in the corn oil-fed mice (25.1 days vs. 33.7 days in the fish oil-fed group). Peak severity score was lower in fish oil-fed mice (6.7 vs 9.8 in the corn oil group). Ultimately 93% of corn oil-fed mice developed arthritis compared with 69% of fish oil-fed mice. By all criteria used (incidence, severity, peak severity, time of onset) fish oil-fed mice were less susceptible to the disease than corn oil-fed mice. Macrophages from the mice fed fish oil produced about half the amount of eicosanoids as those from the corn oil-fed mice [28].

A number of studies have now been performed investigating the biochemical and clinical impact of fish oil in RA; these are summarised in Table 3. These studies have used between 1 and 7.1 g EPA plus DHA per day, provided for 12 and

Table 3. Summary of the trials of fish oil in RA

Duration (weeks)	EPA + DHA (g/day)	Significant improvements in	Reference
12	1.8 + 1.2	Number of tender joints; duration of morning stiffness	29
14	2.7 + 1.8	Number of tender joints; Number of swollen joints; Time to fatigue; Doctor's global assessment	30
12	3.2 + 2.0	Number of tender joints; Grip strength	31
24	1.7 + 1.2	In both groups: Number of tender joints; Number of swollen joints; Grip strength; Doctor's global assessment	32
	or 3.5 + 2.4	In high dose group only: duration of morning stiffness	
12	2.0 + 1.3	Number of swollen joints; Joint pain index	33
12	2.0 + 1.3	Number of swollen joints; Duration of morning stiffness	34
24	1.8 + 1.2	Number and severity of tender joints; Doctor's global assessment; Use of NSAIDs	35
16	3.8 + 2	Number and severity of tender joints; Duration of morning stiffness	36
12	2.0 + 1.2	Number of tender joints; Duration of morning stiffness	37
52	1.7 + 1.1	Use of NSAIDs	38
52	0.8 + 0.2 or 1.7 + 0.4	Doctor's pain assessment; Patient's global assessment; Use of NSAIDs and/or SAARDs	39
26 to 30	4.6 + 2.5	Number of tender joints; Duration of moring stiffness; Doctor's assessment of pain; Doctor's global assessment; Patient's global assessment	40

52 weeks (see Table 3 for details). The amounts of EPA plus DHA used in these studies would equate to between 3 and 21 g of fish oil per day i.e. between 3 and 21 standard 1 g fish oil capsules. Treating RA patients with fish oil led to decreased LTB_4 production by stimulated neutrophils [29–31, 34] and monocytes [31, 32]. Surprisingly the neutrophil chemotactic response is significantly impaired in RA patients [41, 42]; this was shown to be due to marked down-regulation of the LTB_4 receptor and subsequent reduced signalling through this receptor [42]. Feeding fish oil to RA patients up-regulated LTB_4 receptor expression on neutrophils and increased neutrophil chemotaxis towards LTB_4 [42]. In this respect the effect of fish oil was to make neutrophils respond more like those from subjects who did not have RA. A fish oil-induced reduction in IL-1, but not TNF-α or IL-2, production by monocytes from RA patients has been reported [32]. Fish oil lowered circulating C-reactive protein concentration in RA patients [27]. Thus, in RA patients fish oil appears to exert some anti-inflammatory effects (lowered LTB_4, IL-1 and C-reactive protein production), suggesting that it might bring about clinical improvements.

A variety of clinical outcome measures have been monitored in the trials of fish oil in RA (see Table 3). Each study has reported improvements after fish oil, including reduced duration of morning stiffness, reduced number of tender or swollen joints, reduced joint pain, reduced time to fatigue, and increased grip strength (Table 3). In eleven studies fish oil resulted in an improvement in at least two clinical measures, and in four studies there was improvement in at least four clinical outcomes (Table 3). Decreased joint tenderness was reported in nine studies (Table 3). Assessments made by the patient and/or the doctor indicated decreased disease activity in several studies (Table 3). Normal medication was continued during the fish oil supplementation period in most of these studies, although in three of the studies patients were free to change their use of NSAIDs as required [35, 38, 39]. In each of these three studies there was a significant reduction in the use of NSAIDs while patients were consuming fish oil (Table 3). In two other studies cessation of use of NSAIDs was part of the protocol [36, 40] and the ability of patients to endure this suggests an NSAID-sparing effect. Thus, fish oil appears to induce significant clinical improvements in patients with RA and may lead to decreased use of NSAIDs. A meta-analysis of ten of these studies which were randomised and placebo-controlled has been performed [43]. This confirmed significant improvements in the number of tender/ painful joints and in morning stiffness after 3 months of fish oil treatment.

12.8 Conclusions and Comments

The production of arachidonic acid-derived pro-inflammatory eicosanoids such as PGE_2 and LTB_4 is markedly reduced by feeding diets rich in fish oil. Furthermore, inclusion of fish oil in the diet significantly reduces the movement of leukocytes towards chemotactic agents and the production of pro-inflammatory cytokines by monocytes, macrophages and T lymphocytes. Long chain *n-3* fatty acids also appear to reduce adhesion molecule expression and thus might influence the movement of leukocytes into sites of inflammation. Several studies indicate a reduction of major histocompatibility class II expression on antigen presenting cells following fish oil feeding; this would suggest a diminished ability to present antigen. Some studies show that fish oil decreases generation of reactive oxygen species. Although some of the effects of fish oil may be brought about by modulation of the amount and types of eicosanoids made, it is likely that these fatty acids can also elicit their effects by eicosanoid-independent mechanisms. These effects suggest that fish oil may be of use as a therapy for chronic inflammatory disorders such as RA. Trials of fish oil in RA have shown significant improvements in a variety of clinical outcomes. The effectiveness of fish oil might however have been underestimated because in most studies patients have continued with existing drug therapies (Table 3) and because the intake of *n*–6 fatty acids from the diet has not been modified; it is possible that *n-3* fatty acids might be more effectively incorporated into immune cells if *n*–6 fatty acid intake is lowered. On the other hand, the elongation product of linoleic acid, γ-linolenic acid, also has anti-inflammatory effects and has been used alone and in combination with fish oil with some success in RA [see 44, 45 for reviews of the use of γ-linolenic acid in RA]. There have been no detailed studies of the dose-response relationship between EPA plus DHA and clinical improvement in RA. One study which included more than a single dose of EPA plus DHA [32], found that both doses (2.9 and 5.9 g EPA plus DHA per day) were equally as effective at bringing about clinical improvements. However, the improvements became statistically significant sooner in the high dose group than in the low dose group (12 weeks vs. 18 or 24 weeks) [32]. It is not known what the minimum dose required to bring about a range of clinical improvements is, although most studies have used about 3.3 g EPA plus DHA per day. It is not clear what the maximum effective dose of EPA plus DHA is, although the study of Kremer et al. [32] would suggest that a lower dose can be as effective as a high one but will take longer to exert its effects. The potential role of the precursor of EPA, α-linolenic acid, in RA has not been investigated. If α-linolenic acid were to be effective it would most likely need to be converted to EPA. In humans this conversion is not efficient, meaning that large does of α-linolenic acid would be required to affect immunological responses. Caughey et al. [46] have shown that dietary α-linolenic acid can decrease *ex vivo* TNF-α and IL-1β production by monocytes from healthy volunteers, but 13.7 g α-linolenic acid per day for four weeks, approximately 10-times habitual intake, was only about 30% as effective as 2.7 g EPA plus DHA.

12.9 References

1. Report of the British Nutrition Foundation's Task Force. *Unsaturated Fatty Acids: Nutritional and Physiological Significance.* London: Chapman & Hall, 1992
2. British Nutrition Foundation. *n-3 Fatty Acids and Health.* London: British Nutrition Foundation, 1999
3. Mann NJ, Johnson LG, Warrick GE, Sinclair AJ. The arachidonic acid content of the Australian diet is lower than previously estimated. *J Nutr* 1995; 125: 2528–2535

4. Jonnalagadda SS, Egan SK, Heimbach JT, Harris SS, Kris-Etherton PM. Fatty acid consumption pattern of Americans: 1987–1988 USDA Nationwide Food Consumption Survey. *Nutr Res* 1999; 15: 1767–1781
5. Sinclair AJ, O'Dea K. The significance of arachidonic acid in hunter-gatherer diets: implications for the contemporary Western diet. *J Food Lipids* 1993; 1: 143–157
6. Grimble RF. Interaction between nutrients, pro-inflammatory cytokines and inflammation. *Clin Sci* 1996; 91: 121–130
7. Wolfe AM. The epidemiology of rheumatoid arthritis. A review. *Bull Rheum Dis* 1968; 19: 518–532
8. MacGregor A, Ollier W, Thompson W, Jawaheer D, Silman A. HLA-DRB1 0401/0404 genotype and rheumatoid arthritis: Increased association in men, young age at onset, and disease severity. *J Rheumatol* 1995; 22: 1030–1036
9. Firestein GS, Zvaifler NJ. How important are T cells in chronic rheumatoid synovitis? *Arth Rheum* 1990; 33: 768–773
10. Feldmann M, Brennan FM, Maini RN. Role of cytokines in rheumatoid arthritis. *Annu Rev Immunol* 1996; 14: 397–440
11. Sano H, Hla T, Maier JAM et al. In vivo cyclooxygenase expression in synovial tissues of patients with rheumatoid arthritis and osteoarthritis and rats with adjuvant and streptococcal cell wall arthritis. *J Clin Invest* 1992; 89:97–108
12. Sperling RI. Eicosanoids in rheumatoid arthritis. *Rheumat Dis Clin N Amer* 1995; 21: 741–758
13. Mehindate K, Al-Daccak R, Dayer JM. Superantigen-induced collagenase gene expression in human IFN-γ-treated fibroblast-like synoviocytes involves prostaglandin E_2. *J Immunol* 1995; 155: 3570–3577
14. Robinson DR, Tashjian AH, Levine L. Prostaglandin E_2 induced bone resorption by rheumatoid synovia. A model of bone destruction in RA. *J Clin Invest* 1975; 56:1181–1187
15. Lee TH, Hoover RL, Williams JD, Sperling RI et al. Effects of dietary enrichment with EPA and DHA on *in vitro* neutrophil and monocyte leukotriene generation and neutrophil function. *New Engl J Med* 1985; 312: 1217–1224
16. Chapkin RS, Hubbard NE, Erickson KL. 5-Series peptido-leukotriene synthesis in mouse peritoneal macrophages: modulation by dietary n-3 fatty acids. *Biochem Biophys Res Commun* 1991; 171: 764–769
17. Lee TH, Mencia-Huerta J-M, Shih C, Corey EJ, Austen KF. Characterization and biological properties of 5,12-dihydroxy derivatives of EPA, including LTB_5 and the double lipoxygenase product. *J Biol Chem* 1984; 259: 2383–2389
18. Kragballe K, Voorhees JJ, Goetzl EJ. Inhibition by leukotriene B_5 of leukotriene B_4-induced activation of human keratinocytes and neutrophils. *J Invest Dermatol* 1987; 88: 555–558
19. Kinsella JE, Lokesh B, Broughton S, Whelan J. Dietary polyunsaturated fatty acids and eicosanoids: potential effects on the modulation of inflammatory and immune cells: An overview. *Nutrition* 1990; 6: 24–44
20. Calder PC. Effects of fatty acids and dietary lipids on cells of the immune system. *Proc Nutr Soc* 1996; 55: 127–150
21. Blok WL, Katan MB, van der Meer JWM. Modulation of inflammation and cytokine production by dietary (n-3) fatty acids. *J Nutr* 1996; 126: 1515–1533
22. Calder PC. N-3 polyunsaturated fatty acids and cytokine production in health and disease. *Ann Nutr Metab* 1997; 4: 203–234
23. Yaqoob P. Lipids and the immune response. *Curr Opin Clin Nutr Metab Care* 1998; 1: 153–161
24. Alexander JW. Immunonutrition: The role of ω-3 fatty acids. *Nutrition* 1998; 14: 627–633
25. Miles EA, Calder PC. Modulation of immune function by dietary fatty acids. *Proc Nutr Soc* 1998; 57: 277–92
26. Calder PC. Dietary fatty acids and lymphocyte functions. *Proc Nutr Soc* 1998; 57: 487–502

27. Calder PC. n-3 Polyunsaturated fatty acids and mononuclear phagocyte function. In: Kremer J (ed) *Medicinal Fatty Acids in Inflammation*. Basel: Birkhauser Verlag, pp 1–27, 1998
28. Leslie CA, Gonnerman WA, Ullman MD, Hayes KC, Franzblau C, Cathcart ES. Dietary fish oil modulates macrophage fatty acids and decreases arthritis susceptibility in mice. *J Exp Med* 1985; 162: 1336–1349
29. Kremer JM, Bigaouette J, Michalek AV et al. Effects of manipulation of dietary fatty acids on clinical manifestations of rheumatoid arthritis. *Lancet* 1985; i: 184–187
30. Kremer JM, Jubiz W, Michalek A et al. Fish-oil fatty acid supplementation in active rheumatoid arthritis. A double-blinded, controlled cross-over study. *Ann Intern Med* 1987; 106: 497–502
31. Cleland LG, French JK, Betts WH, Murphy GA, Elliot MJ. Clinical and biochemical effects of dietary fish oil supplements in rheumatoid arthritis. *J Rheumatol* 1988; 15: 1471–1475
32. Kremer JM, Lawrence DA, Jubiz W et al. Dietary fish oil and olive oil supplementation in patients with rheumatoid arthritis. Clinical and immunologic findings. *Arth Rheum* 1990; 33: 810–820
33. Tulleken JE, Limburg PC, Muskiet FAJ, van Rijswijk MH. Vitamin E status during dietary fish oil supplementation in rheumatoid arthritis. *Arth Rheum* 1990; 33: 1416–1419
34. Van der Tempel H, Tulleken JE, Limburg PC, Muskiet FAJ, van Rijswijk MH. Effects of fish oil supplementation in rheumatoid arthritis. *Ann Rheum Dis* 1990; 49: 76–80
35. Skoldstam L, Borjesson O, Kjallman A, Seiving B, Akesson B. Effect of six months of fish oil supplementation in stable rheumatoid arthritis: a double-blind, controlled study. *Scand J Rheumatol* 1992; 21: 178–185
36. Kjeldsen-Kragh J, Lund JA, Riise T et al. Dietary n-3 fatty acid supplementation and naproxen treatment in patients with rheumatoid arthritis. *J Rheumatol* 1992; 19: 1531–536
37. Nielsen GL, Faarvang KL, Thomsen BS et al. The effect of dietary supplementation with n-3 polyunsaturated fatty acids in patients with rheumatoid arthritis: a randomised, double blind trial. *Eur J Clin Invest* 1992; 22: 687–691
38. Lau CS, Morley KD, Belch JJF. Effects of fish oil supplementation on non-steroidal anti-inflammatory drug requirement in patients with mild rheumatoid arthritis. *Brit J Rheumatol* 1993; 32: 982–989
39. Geusens P, Wouters C, Nijs J, Jiang Y, Dequeker J. Long-term effect of omega-3 fatty acid supplementation in active rheumatoid arthritis. *Arth Rheum* 1994; 37: 824–829
40. Kremer JM, Lawrence DA, Petrillo GF et al. The effect of high dose fish oil on rheumatoid arthritis after stopping NSAIDs: clinical and immune correlates in patients with rheumatoid arthritis. *Arth Rheum* 1995; 38: 1107–1114
41. Sperling RI, Weinblatt M, Robin J-L et al. Effects of dietary supplementation with marine fish oil on leukocyte lipid mediator generation and function in rheumatoid arthritis. *Arth Rheum* 1987; 30: 988–997
42. Sperling RI, Sohl P, Chen ZS, Lewis-Mannion M, Austen KF, Robinson DR. Suppressed chemotactic responsiveness of PMN from patients with RA is due to downregulated receptor number and signalling. *Arth Rheum* 1993; 36: S244
43. Fortin PR, Lew RA, Liang MH et al. Validation of a meta-analysis: the effects of fish oil in rheumatoid arthritis. *J Clin Epidemiol* 1995; 48: 1379–1390
44. Zurier RB. Gammalinolenic acid treatment of rheumatoid arthritis. In: Kremer J (ed) *Medicinal Fatty Acids in Inflammation*. Basel: Birkhauser Verlag, pp 29–43, 1998
45. Belch JJF, Muir A. *n*–6 and *n-3* Essential fatty acids in rheumatoid arthritis and other rheumatic conditions. *Proc Nutr Soc* 1998; 57: 563–569
46. Caughey GE, Mantzioris E, Gibson RA, Cleland LG, James MJ. The effect on human tumor necrosis factor α and interleukin 1 β production of diets enriched in n-3 fatty acids from vegetable oil or fish oil. *Am J Clin Nutr* 1996; 63: 116–122